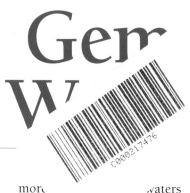

# Ger
## W

more vaters
for th eatments

## Michael Gienger
## Joachim Goebel

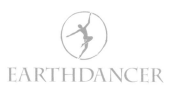

EARTHDANCER

A FINDHORN PRESS IMPRINT

*Gem Water*
Michael Gienger/Joachim Goebel
With photographs by Ines Blersch

Fourth Edition 2014

This English edition © 2007 Earthdancer GmbH
English translation © 2007 Astrid Mick
Editorial: JMS Books

Originally published in German as *Wassersteine*
World © 2006 Neue Erde GmbH, Saarbruecken, Germany

All rights reserved.

Title page:
Photo: Ines Blersch
Design: Dragon Design UK

Typeset and graphics:
Dragon Design UK
Set in News Gothic

Total Production: Midas Printing

Printed and bound in China

ISBN 978-1-84409-131-7

Published by Earthdancer GmbH, an imprint of:
Findhorn Press, 117-121 High Street, Forres, IV36 1AB, Scotland
www.earthdancer.co.uk . www.findhornpress.com

FSC
MIX
Paper from responsible sources
FSC® C011223
www.fsc.org

# Contents

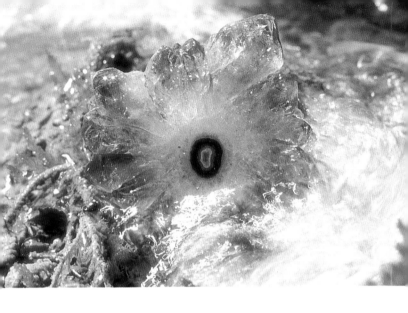

## The gem water handbook

Following the publication of their first book, *Edelsteinwasser*, (published in German, by Neue Erde 2006) and in the wake of the number of crystals used for gem water having doubled in the course of just one year, the authors Michael Gienger and Joachim Goebel soon realized that they needed to write a second volume. Benefiting from the authors' recent experiences with new ways of using gem water as a healing remedy, this new book forms an ideal introduction to the subject. It explains the basic principles and the different methods of making gem water and gives tried and tested gem water 'recipes', along with a directory of the best crystals to use and their different effects.

It is becoming apparent that, when used in gem water preparations, healing crystals do not have quite the same effects as when they are applied or worn externally as gems or stones. Water as a medium influences the crystals and the effects they produce. It seems that the nature of water causes a selection process to take place. This book therefore does not describe all the known effects of the healing crystals themselves, but mainly their therapeutic effects when combined with water. It forms an essential guide to the use of gem water as a healing remedy, for yourself or for others.

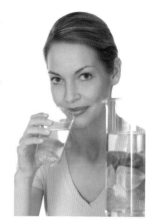

Since no other branch of crystal healing is currently developing at quite such speed, it is impossible to produce a book at the current time that is guaranteed to be complete, but the authors are keen to make their knowledge and experience available to anyone interested in the subject – so that further effects can be researched and uses developed that can be of benefit to everyone.

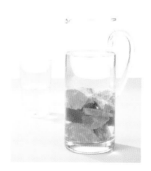

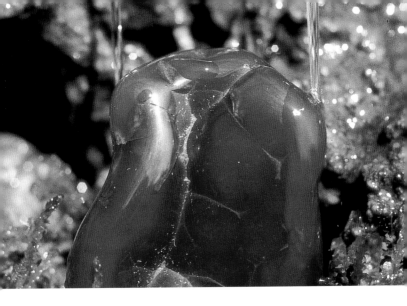

## *Basic principles of gem water application*

### Mineral water and gem water

During the production of gem water, information contained in the rocks, minerals and crystals that are used is transferred to the water. When gem water is taken internally or applied externally it therefore has similar effects to when the crystals themselves are used in healing. Crucially, however, it is not any physical substance from the crystal that is transferred to the water – the crystal does not dissolve in it – it is solely energy from the crystal that is conveyed. Gem waters are there-fore 'healing aids and applications', similar to homeopathic remedies or Bach flower essences. Their effectiveness relies on the information contained in the gem water, not in the water or crystal itself.

This is the difference between gem waters and mineral waters, by which we normally mean water that is enriched by traces of minerals.

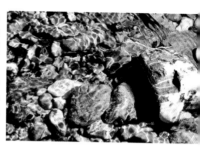

Mineral water can also be taken as a healing remedy. For example, the mineral water from some springs is used to treat eye problems, kidney problems, digestive disturbances, rheumatism and many other complaints. Which mineral waters really do offer some health benefits and which do not is, however, something over which experts disagree – but it is always the type and amount of minerals dissolved in the water and their biochemical effects that is debated. By contrast, gem waters are, if possible, created in such a way that no minerals, or as few as possible, are dissolved in the water. Ideally, the water does not undergo any physical changes, but despite this the water *is* altered, as most people can tell from the taste. Depending on the crystal and water used, the water appears softer, fresher, and sometimes even tastier. The growth of bacteria in gem water is also slowed, so the water does not become stale so quickly, as demonstrated in a study carried out at the Hygiene Consultation Centre Pestel in Schwäbisch-Gmünd (Germany). Water that was left standing in the open, and which had been energized with Quartz, remained bacteria-free for several weeks.

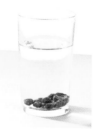

*'Gem water', the term used to describe water that has been informed by crystals, is distinct from 'mineral water' – naturally occurring water containing minerals – which, because of its biochemical effect, is used as a therapeutic aid.*

We therefore use the term 'gem water' even if we use 'ordinary' minerals or rocks to inform the water.

## Gem water as drinking water

We can achieve two goals in making gem water – we can improve the quality of our drinking water (without intending to give it any particular effect), but we can also create a therapeutic remedy with a very specific effect. Only very few crystals can actually be used simply to improve the quality of drinking water, as most transfer very specific information and therefore have a corresponding specific effect. For example, only Clear Quartz is sufficiently neutral to be considered 'unspecific'. The properties of Clear Quartz, such as freshness, clarity, vitality and energy, resemble the very essence of those properties we normally associate with water, to the extent that the Greek origin of the name *krystallos* (meaning 'ice') is particularly appropriate. Clear Quartz supports water's inherent quality as a pure, clear source of life.

Amethyst and Rose Quartz, closely related, are often added to Clear Quartz to create a 'basic mixture'; they are not only clearly more colourful in their appearance, but also in their effects. Although their effects are normally regarded as very pleasant – after all, who does not want to experience feelings of 'alertness, consciousness and inner peace' (Amethyst) or 'sensuality, sensitivity to the world and liveliness' (Rose Quartz) – the water they create is not neutral, but rather a beneficial 'well-being drink'.

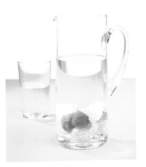

The advantage of gem waters made with these types of quartz is that you can use them over periods of several months, if you wish, so we can justifiably refer to Amethyst, Rose Quartz and Clear Quartz as 'crystals for improving drinking water'.

However, we must be careful not to allow any misunderstandings to arise. It would quite simply be wrong to suggest that placing crystals in water could make purifying water with filters or improving its quality through swirling unnecessary. Gems can only transfer information to the water – they cannot remove any harmful or damaging substances from it. This therefore means that placing crystals in water cannot replace any system of water purification or revitalization. Crystals such as Amethyst, Clear Quartz and Rose Quartz can 'improve' drinking water only by helping to make it taste better, keep fresh for longer (by inhibiting the growth of bacteria, see above), and make the water easier for the body to absorb.

## Gem water for healing

Creating gem water as an aid to healing is something quite different from the process of treating drinking water. In the case of the former the crucial aim is to improve our health (or someone else's) rather than to improve the quality of the water. Gem water created for healing is essentially a remedy and should therefore not be drunk on a regular basis, but rather be taken in specific doses or applied externally.

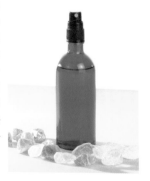

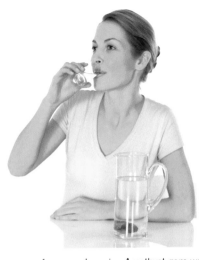

**Applying gem water externally:** When used externally, gem water may have several advantages over using the crystals themselves. Very often a crystal simply cannot physically be applied where it is needed, or it may simply be too small to cover the area required. Gem water, on the other hand, can be generously applied with cotton wool, or as a compress, or you can even bathe in it! According to the medieval naturalist Hildegard von Bingen, traditional applications include, for example, using Amethyst gem water as a facial and skin tonic. Gem water prepared with Aventurine and Prase can be applied topically for sunburn and minor burns. Excellent gem water combinations prepared with Rhodonite or Mookaite can, for example, be sprayed with care onto open wounds from a small, sterile spray bottle. This method of applying gem water is particularly suitable for grazes, where the crystals themselves cannot be applied directly. Gem water can also be added to bath water. In this case it should be prepared over a longer period to obtain a particularly concentrated preparation, which you can then add to the water, ideally just before you climb into the bath. When you use gem water and other bath additives (see page 62), you can create a really wonderful feeling of well-being.

**Using gem water internally:** You can take gem water internally as a naturopathic or therapeutic remedy for physical or emotional problems, following the same rules as for any similar healing treatment.

*1. It is extremely important to use the correct crystals. When crystals are worn externally, they can obviously be removed easily if any adverse reactions are experienced; however, when gem water is taken internally, you are inevitably subjected to its effects, as with any other healing remedy taken internally. This is why externally applied crystals are much more suitable for use if you are in any doubt as to how you will react to them; it is even more important when using gem water internally to be cautious if there is any uncertainty as to the outcome, and to seek expert advice.*

*2. It is important to use the right dose, as some gem waters have such a strong effect that they should be taken only in shot glass measures (2 tablespoons/20–30 ml). Chrysoprase gem water is a good example of one that must only be taken in specific small quantities, for detoxification, while other types of gem water can be taken in larger quantities, such as Diamond gem water taken after a stroke. See the chapter called 'Quantity and intensity' (page 36).*

*3. The use of gem water should also be restricted in the case of serious physical ailments, severe mental problems, during pregnancy, or during homeopathic treatment. Always discuss using gem water in such cases with the appropriate doctors or therapists. See also the chapter called 'Effects and applications'.*

Providing you follow these rules, gem water makes a very successful healing treatment, as both traditional and modern usage has proved.

## Quality of the water

The purer the water (the fewer substances dissolved in it), the less 'pre-programmed' it will be and therefore the better it can absorb information from the crystals. Applying high pressure to the water – of the kind that is used to control the flow of water through the household mains supply – is detrimental to the absorption. It also goes without saying that the water you use should not contain any harmful substances.

The following waters are good for producing gem water:

- *Water (containing a minimum amount of minerals) derived from sources of granite, sandstone and volcanic rock.*
- *Bottled water (containing a minimum amount of minerals) from glass bottles: a mineral content of less than 200mg/l is ideal; less than 500mg/l is also suitable (just add up the mineral values indicated on the label).*
- *Mains water that has been passed through an activated carbon block filter.*
- *Mains water that has been purified through a reverse osmosis system\*.*
- *Water that has been purified through filtration (carbon filter/ reverse osmosis) and made 'information free' through colloidation, a type of intensive whirling*

Not suitable for producing gem water:

- *Mineral-rich spring or mains water: you can use water with a mineral content below 1000mg/l but only to a degree; if the mineral content is any higher, the water is verging on not being able to absorb any information. This includes very hard water.*
- *Water from plastic bottles: the substances from which plastic bottles are made release chemical substances (softeners) into water, which is why drinking water from them is not recommended.*
- *Unfiltered mains water: in particular, it is the pressure under which the water is pumped through the system that makes it less able to absorb information. This, in turn, means that the water will quickly lose the information from the crystals again.*

\* As water purified by reverse osmosis is slightly acidic and may remove minerals from the body, purification installations containing Calcite filters that increase the pH of acidic water should be used. If this water is to be used on a long-term basis, it is important to make sure that your diet contains sufficient minerals.

- *Water filtered by non-solid carbon filters; these filters have no proven purification effect, and can, if they are used for longer periods, even release toxic substances back into the water.*

## Crystal quality

The better the quality of the crystals used, the better the quality of the resulting gem water. So it is a good idea to take the following into account when choosing crystals:

**Signs of good quality:** For the best results, choose crystals that display their characteristic natural properties to the full. Depending on the type of crystal, look out for colour, markings, purity, transparency, luminescence and brilliance and, in some cases, the shape of the crystal, magnetism and optical effects.

**Purity:** The crystals used should be completely natural and not have been treated in any way. Crystals are sometimes treated (such as irradiated, heated; dyed; impregnated with artificial resin), which will change the effects and effectiveness of the crystals. Synthetic crystals will also display different properties from their natural equivalents, but obviously do not use imitation crystals for producing gem water.

**Suitable types of crystal:** Crystals and raw gemstones (even fragments) are among the best types, but they should all be free of the matrix in order to avoid contaminating the water or altering the effects of the crystals. To reduce the risk of broken fragments getting into the water, polished crystals (without settings) as well as pre-tumbled or tumbled 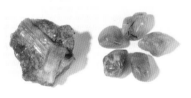 crystals, can be used. In the tumbling process, raw crystals are placed in large polishing tumblers that revolve like washing machines, only much more slowly. They mimic the rolling action of crystals in running water in nature, producing rounded pebble shapes out of jagged crystals. If crystals are tumbled for a short time only, just to break off sharp edges and remove sharp fragments, they are known as 'pre-tumbled' crystals. If the tumbling is carried out for longer, until the crystals become smooth and rounded, they are known simply as 'tumbled'.

**No wax or oil:** Decorative crystals that are used externally, tumbled crystals and even some raw crystals are often waxed or oiled, and you should avoid using these for preparing gem water, especially if they are going to be placed directly in water. These types of crystal are only suitable for 'indirect' methods of preparation, during which there is no contact between the water and the crystals, and even then the oil and wax on the crystals surfaces may result in changes in their effect on water.

**Size and surface area:** When placing the crystals directly in water, as well as when using the boiling and evaporation methods, (see 'Preparation methods', page 28), the contact area between the crystal and the water will determine the intensity of the gem water that is created. The larger the area of contact between the crystals and the water, the faster the information will be absorbed and the more intense the gem water produced within a short time. So, several smaller crystals have a more intense effect than a smaller number of larger ones, just as crystals with rough surfaces have a more intense effect than crystals that are naturally smooth or highly polished.

Generally suitable for producing gem water:
- *Crystals and raw gemstones (including fragments) without attached matrix.*
- *Pre-tumbled or tumbled crystals, unwaxed crystals.*
- *Polished gems without settings.*

<u>Not</u> suitable for placing in water directly, but only for indirect preparation methods (test tube method; conducting with crystals) and with certain restrictions.

- *Crystals and raw crystals with matrix.*
- *Waxed and oiled crystals.*
- *Toxic crystals (please see 'Important – some crystals can be toxic!' below).*

Not suitable for producing gem water:

- *Irradiated, heated, dyed crystals, and crystals impregnated with artificial resins.*
- *Synthetic crystals and imitations.*
- *Joined crystals (twins and triplets).*

Important – some crystals can be toxic!

Some healing crystals that can be used in external applications without a qualm may release toxic substances if they are placed directly in water, or if they are used in the boiling and evaporation methods (see 'Preparation methods', page 28). Therefore, these crystals should never be used for those preparation methods. For these types of crystals we recommend the 'indirect' preparation methods, such as the test tube method or the method of conducting information with crystals, which avoid direct contact between the water and the crystal.

The following list is a guide to those healing crystals that are not suitable for placing directly in water. However, since new crystals are constantly being introduced to the market, we cannot guarantee that this list is complete. When in doubt, please always follow these guidelines:

*1. Crystals not listed as bona fide healing crystals by authenticated sources should never be placed in drinking water or used internally as healing remedies.*

*2. More detailed information about healing crystals that may release toxic substances can be found in the book by Gienger/Goebel, 'Edelsteinwasser'. Internet web-pages, www.edelstein-wasser.de and www.steinheilkunde.ev.de will also provide regular up-dated information on the subject.*

*3. When in doubt, only use those methods in which the crystals are not placed directly in water to produce gem water.*

## Crystals that are NOT suitable for placing in water:

**Alunite (Alum):** Non toxic but soluble in water.

**Anglesite:** Toxic and slightly soluble in water.

**Arsenopyrite:** Potentially toxic.

**Atacamite:** Potentially harmful.

**Azurite:** Harmful.

**Azurite-Malachite:** Harmful.

**Azurite-Pseudomalachite:** Harmful.

**Bunsenite:** Toxic; allergen; avoid skin contact.

**Calomel:** Possibly hazardous to health.

**Cerussite (white lead ore):** Toxic.

**Chalcanthite (copper vitriol):** Harmful; easily soluble in water.

**Cinnabar (Cinnabarite):** Very toxic!

**Cinnabar-Opal:** The cinnabar stored in the opal is toxic.

**Crocoite:** Toxic.

**Cuprite:** Harmful.

**Durangite:** Potentially toxic.

**Eclipse Stone:** Limestone with orpiment, toxic.

**Eilat Stone (Chrysocolla-Malachite-Azurite):** Harmful.

**Erythrite:** Potentially toxic.

**Fiedlerite:** Toxic.

**Fluorite, Antozonite ('stink spar') variety:** Potentially harmful.

**Galenite (Galena):** Toxic and slightly soluble in water.

**Gaspeite:** Harmful; allergen; avoid skin contact.

**Greenockite:** Toxic.

**Halite (rock salt; crystalline salt):** Not toxic in small quantities, but dissolves easily in water.

**Iron-nickel Meteorite:** Harmful; allergen; avoid skin contact.

**Jamesonite:** Potentially toxic.

**Lemon Chrysoprase (nickel magnesite):** Potentially harmful; allergen; avoid skin contact.

**Lopezite:** Very toxic! Hazardous even through skin contact.

**Malachite:** Harmful.

**Millerite (nickel sulphide):** Toxic; allergen; avoid skin contact.

**Minium:** Toxic.

**Nickeline (nickel arsenide):** Toxic; allergen; avoid skin contact.

**Olivenite:** Potentially toxic.

**Orpiment:** Toxic.

**Proustite:** Potentially toxic.

**Psilomelane and Pyrolusite:** Harmful.

**Pyromorphite:** Potentially toxic.

**Rauenthalite:** Toxic.

**Realgar:** Toxic. Store in a dark, securely locked place.

**Scorodite:** Potentially toxic.

**Sphaerocobaltite:** Harmful; allergen; avoid skin contact.

**Stibnite (Antimonite):** Harmful.

**Tetrahedrite:** Potentially harmful.

**Ulexite:** Non toxic but slightly soluble in warm water.

**Valentinite (flower of antimony) and Senarmontite:** Harmful.

**Vanadinite:** Toxic.

**Wulfenite (yellow lead ore):** Potentially toxic.

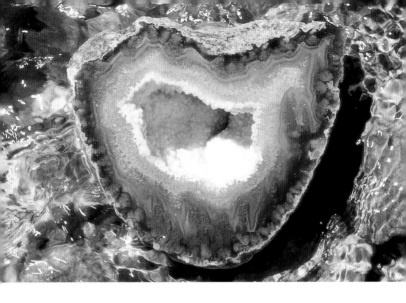

## Making gem water

The preparation methods for gem water differ considerably and are covered in detail in the next chapter. However, the basic methods for preparing and making them are common to all.

### General preparation

You will not need all the equipment or to follow all the steps listed below for every preparation method. If you want to prepare gem water very quickly, then all you need is some water, a glass and the appropriate crystal.

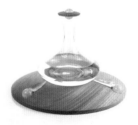

However, if you want to produce high-quality gem water and possibly store it for some time, you should make sure that each step is carried out carefully. So, first of all, make sure that you have the following items to hand:

## Checklist of materials

### General:

- A glass jug of water that will absorb information (see page 22).
- A plain glass container for preparing the gem water (the glass should be colourless and, if possible, not bear any inscriptions or engravings, etc).
- Your selected crystals.
- A soft bristle brush for cleansing the crystals.
- High-percentage rubbing alcohol for sterilizing.
- A clean, soft cloth for applying the rubbing alcohol.
- An Amethyst geode or cluster, or a 'salt dish' (see page 21) for the energetic cleansing of the crystals.
- Sterilized wooden tongs, tweezers or similar for handling cleansed crystals.
- A clean, sterilized tea strainer or a glass funnel lined with filter paper for decanting the gem water.
- A storage bottle (violet or blue glass is best).
- Brandy (only required for long-term storage).
- A cloth for drying the crystals.

### For special preparation methods:

- A quartz glass test tube for the test tube method
- An enamel saucepan for the boiling method or the 'evaporation' method.
- Wooden sticks or wooden tongs for placing the crystals in the container for the 'evaporation' method.
- Clear Quartz or Laser Wand Quartz Crystal are best for 'conducting information'.
- Crystal slices.
- Crystal dishes.

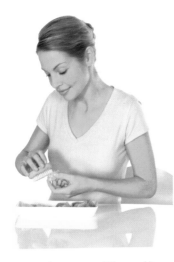

## Cleansing the crystals

Before you can begin making the gem water, you must first cleanse the crystals, which can take some time, so remember to plan ahead for this. Thoroughly cleansing the crystal itself is a good idea, especially if your crystals are new or they have not been used for a long time, and after this the 'energy' of the crystals must also be cleansed, as follows:

The first step in the cleansing process is **to brush** the crystals vigorously. If they are very dirty use a little washing-up liquid – preferably an ecological brand. Afterwards, rinse the crystal thoroughly under cold running water.

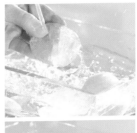

**Disinfecting** with rubbing alcohol helps combat the growth of bacteria while the crystals are in the water. However, as the alcohol will reduce the water's ability to absorb information, the crystals should be rinsed thoroughly under cold, running water afterwards. As you will be touching the crystals with your hands once the energetic cleansing process is complete, you should also wash your hands thoroughly and, if necessary, use an antibacterial hand-wash.

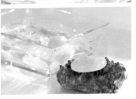

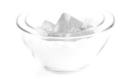

**Energetic cleansing** involves purifying the crystals under cold, running water (so that any energy previously absorbed can be discharged), followed by cleansing with an Amethyst geode or cluster, to ensure any foreign information that has been absorbed is completely removed. As this takes some time, you should start the process of cleansing the crystals well in advance of preparing the gem water.

**To purify** a crystal, hold it under cold, running water for about a minute while rubbing it vigorously with your thumb. After a while, the surface of the crystal will start to feel different and your thumb will not slide across it so easily. When this happens you will know that the purification is complete.

To make absolutely sure that the crystals **have been cleansed of any remaining foreign information** before you make your gem water, place the purified crystals on the points of an Amethyst geode or a piece of Amethyst cluster for at least two hours, but preferably longer – eight to twelve hours would be even better. The energetic radiation of the Amethyst points will remove any foreign information.

*It is often very difficult to remove foreign information from crystals that have been exposed to extreme energetic stress. These crystals can be cleansed quickly and thoroughly by placing them in a 'salt dish'. Place some coarse, untreated rock salt in a shallow glass bowl and then place another, empty bowl on top of the salt. Place your crystals in this second bowl and leave them for between ten minutes and two hours. Don't leave them in the salt dish any longer or they will become energetically depleted and lose their effectiveness.*

Don't cleanse too many crystals at a time on a piece of Amethyst cluster or in a salt dish. The individual crystals need to be spaced a few centimetres apart from each other. If you are using salt for cleansing, use a separate salt dish for each type of crystal and discard the salt once the crystal has been cleansed.

In order to be as careful as possible, you should no longer touch the crystals with your bare hands – instead use small wooden tongs, a pair of tweezers, or something similar, depending on the size of the crystals.

## Composing yourself

Once the crystals have been cleansed, you need a suitable place in which to prepare your gem water. A pleasant ambience and a good, stress-free environment are important, as information from the surrounding area will also be absorbed by the water. Make sure you have all your equipment and the cleansed crystals to hand, ready for the following steps (depending on the healing process chosen). Then, allow yourself just a few moments to focus your thoughts calmly on what you are about to do, as gem water is best prepared when you are in a relaxed frame of mind and can give it your full attention.

## Water and containers

First, place the water that you have chosen to use in a very clean glass container. As washing-up liquid and similar substances are not good for gem water, make sure you have rinsed the container extremely well under hot running water first. Ideally, for the final rinse you should use a little of the water that you are going to use to make the gem water.

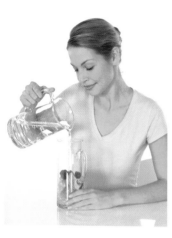

### Preparing the gem water

Now that the initial preparation is complete, you can begin making the gem water. With most of the preparation methods, it makes sense to position the crystals first and then to pour the water into the container, or, as in the case of the conduction method, for example, to position the crystals around the container and then to pour in the water. This ensures that you can make any necessary adjustment to the crystals without making the water impure. The individual preparation methods are explained in detail in the chapter 'Preparation methods', page 28.

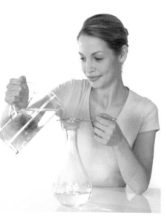

### Decanting the gem water

When you decant the gem water, make sure that no tiny fragments of crystal that might have broken off remain in the water. Fragments of colourless, clear crystals, such as Clear Quartz, are usually extremely hard to detect, so we recommend that you:

- pour the gem water through a clean, sterilized tea strainer, or
- filter the gem water through filter paper.

If you decide to filter the gem water, to be on the safe side use unbleached coffee filter paper.

Use a thoroughly clean glass funnel (available from pharmacies) to pour the gem water into the storage container, as a plastic or stainless steel funnel will adversely affect the quality of the gem water.

## Storing gem water

Water absorbs information well – but equally can easily lose it again. Gem water is therefore essentially a 'fresh' product with a limited 'shelf life'. Depending on how and where you store the gem water, it will keep in a sealed container for up to a week. Here are some tips on the best way to store it.

Gem water should be stored in a place where you feel comfortable, too – it's a bit like needing a comfortable, stress-free bedroom in order to sleep well. The gem water that you are using at any given time should be kept where you can see it. If it is constantly within sight, it will automatically remind you to drink it or use it on a regular basis.

If you want to keep the gem water for longer than a week, the following will help to improve its 'shelf-life'.

Keep gem water in a **cool, dark place**. The warmer the water, the faster it will lose the information it has stored, and strong light, such as direct sunlight, will have the same effect. By storing the gem water in cool conditions and protected from light, it will keep at least twice as long.

Store gem water in a place that is **free from radiation** – earth rays and electromagnetic fields (electrosmog) will destroy the information in the gems. If necessary, have your home dowsed by an expert (this would be worthwhile in any case, in the interests of your health).

Keep gem water in a **sealed container**. If stored in an open container, it will only retain its effectiveness for a day, so make sure you use sealed bottles. Blue glass is good, but violet glass is even better, as it can protect the gem water from information absorbed from radiation or other influences.

Gem water can be stored in sealed violet-coloured glass bottles for weeks or even months.

Adding good-quality alcohol in a ratio of 1:10 – one part brandy (fruit brandy, or similar) to ten parts gem water – can help preserve the information in the gem water for several months. If you decide to use alcohol, first pour the gem water into the container and then add the alcohol.

## Drying the crystals

Once the gem water has been decanted, the crystals that you used should be cleansed then dried very thoroughly to prevent the growth of germs from algae or bacteria. If you are preparing gem water on a continuous basis, the crystals involved should be cleansed at least every ten days.

## Numbers and quantities

How many crystals will you need to prepare the gem water? There are several factors to take into consideration:

The desired intensity – do you want your gem water to be gently or intensely effective? This will depend upon your own health and constitution – if you have a fairly robust constitution, you could probably take a stronger gem water, but obviously a gentle one would be advisable if you are a little more sensitive. You can adjust the quantities in the table on page 27 – the intensity of the gem water increases significantly according to the number of crystals placed in the water.

*'The more the better' is a saying that should never be applied to gem water. It is very important to use the correct dose, which, in fact, may only need to be very low. If in doubt, therefore, begin with gem water of a lower intensity. If the treatment does not take effect, you can try increasing the intensity of the gem water.*

**Type of crystal:** The type of crystal used is the most important factor when making gem water. If you are using a highly potent stone – such

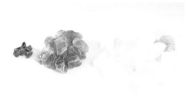

as Diamond, for example – between one and three small raw stones (3–4 mm diameter) per litre of water will be sufficient. In the case of Peridot, which is also potent, three to five raw or tumbled finger-nail-sized gems per litre will be sufficient. With Amethyst, which has a comparatively gentle effect, you can use a whole handful of crystals, while there is theoretically no limit to the number of Clear Quartz crystals you can use.

**Crystal quality:** The quality of the crystals used is also important. A dark-green Aventurine, for example, is more intense than a light-green one. For the dark-green Aventurine, therefore, three or four tumbled gems per litre of gem water will be quite sufficient – whereas you can use a handful for the light-green.

**The preparation method:** The third factor to take into account is the actual method of preparing the gem water. The gentlest methods are those where the glass container of water is placed on a crystal slice, or the crystals are

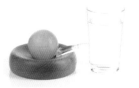

placed directly in the water, or the water is placed in crystal dishes. These methods require the greatest quantity of crystals. The evapora-tion or boiling methods are obviously more intense and so require only half the quantity of crystals. The most intensive method is transferring energy with crystals. You normally only need one crystal for this, regardless of its size. The strength of the gem water is determined by the crystals used, based on their purity, clarity and quality.

**The surface area of the crystal:** In preparation methods where the crystal is in direct contact with the water, the intensity of the gem water is determined by the surface area of the crystals; thus, several smaller crystals will have a greater surface area and therefore a more intense effect than fewer, larger crystals. Similarly, crystals with a rough surface will produce a more intensely effective gem water than naturally smooth crystals or those that have been polished until smooth.

**In conclusion:** With so many factors to take into account, it is not possible to establish a hard and fast rule as to how many crystals should be used for which method, but you can use the following as a rough guide:

**Quantity/Number of healing crystals per litre of gem water**

| | Placed directly in water | Evaporation/ boiling method | Energy transfer with crystals |
|---|---|---|---|
| Highly potent crystals, good quality | individual crystals (1–3 pieces) | individual crystals (1–3 pieces) | just one crystal! |
| Highly potent crystals, medium quality | 5–25g, depending on size* | 5–25g, depending on size* | just one crystal! |
| Very potent crystals of good quality | 25–50g, depending on size* | 10–25g, depending on size* | 1–3 pieces |
| Very potent crystals of medium quality | 50–100g, depending on size* | 25–50g, depending on size* | 1–3 pieces |
| Gentle crystals of good quality | 75–150g, depending on size* | 50–100g, depending on size* | 1–3 pieces, possibly more |
| Gentle crystals of medium quality | 100–200g dep. on size* | 50–100g dep. on size* | 1–3 pieces, possibly more |

* If several crystals of different sizes can be used, the quantities are given in grams.
  Please note: The smaller the individual crystals, the fewer you will need in total. With crystals that are polished smooth (for example, larger tumbled crystals) you can increase the amount.
  Do not use crystals of poor quality, as the gem water produced may not be very effective.

**The categorization of crystal:** The effectiveness of healing crystals and gem waters can be categorized as 'gentle', 'strong' and 'intense', as explained in the chapters on 'Gem water mixtures' (page 41) and 'Index of crystals for gem water preparation' (page 64).

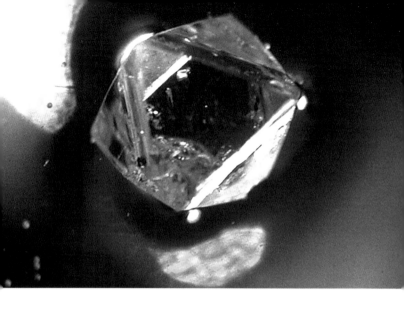

## Preparation methods

There are seven different methods of preparing gem water, each with its own advantages and disadvantages – we have added a note about these after each entry. Generally speaking, none of the processes is better or worse than any of the others. The method you choose depends on how much time you have, the intensity you require and so on.

### Placing crystals directly in water

First cleanse the crystals as described on page 21, then place them directly in the water. The gem water will be ready to use after two to eight hours. You can keep up continuous production by regularly topping up the container with water. However, in this case you should take the crystals out once a week and thoroughly cleanse and dry them, then return them to the water.

**Advantage:** This method of preparation is simple and can be carried out almost anywhere. In an emergency, you could even just use an ordinary drinking glass of water with the crystals.

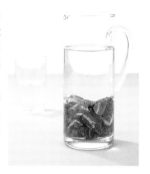

**Disadvantage:** Because the crystals and the water are in direct contact, you must be careful never to use any toxic crystals for this method (see page 15).

## The boiling method

First cleanse the crystals as described on page 21, then place them in cold water, heat slowly to boiling point and boil for five minutes. Leave the crystals in the water until it is completely cool, then decant the gem water into storage bottles.

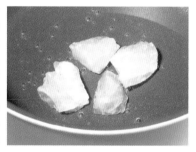

**Advantage:** During boiling, the water will lose almost all the information previously stored in it; then, when it is cooling down, it will absorb new information particularly well. With this method, you can create a very intense gem water in just a short time.

**Disadvantage:** Boiling could damage or even destroy fragile crystals; it could also release toxic substances (see page 15). The only crystals suitable for this method are listed in the 'Index of crystals for gem water preparation' (page 64).

## The evaporation method

Cleanse the crystals as described on page 21, then suspend them for about 30 minutes over an enamel saucepan of gently simmering water, so that the 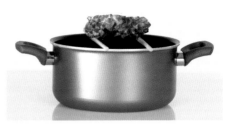 steam condenses on the crystal and drips back into the water. Extract the gem water as soon as it has cooled.

**Advantage:** When it evaporates, water loses any information that has been previously stored in it, so in this method the water absorbs information well, producing a very intense gem water.

**Disadvantage:** Fragile crystals could be damaged or even destroyed with this method, and toxic substances could also be released (see page 15), so you should only use those crystals that are suitable as listed in the 'Index of crystals for gem water preparation' (see page 64).

## The test tube method

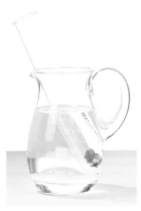

First cleanse the crystals as described on page 21, then place them in a test tube made of pure quartz glass, then stand the test tube in a glass container of water. With this method, you can top up the water in the container and so keep producing the gem water on a continuous basis.

**Advantage:** You can prepare gem water by this method using any type of crystal, even those that are toxic, oiled or waxed so this is the perfect method to use if you have any doubts as to the quality of the crystal.

**Disadvantage:** As there is no direct contact between the crystals and the water, the preparation time will be longer than with other methods.

## Transferring energy from crystals

Energy from crystals that have been thoroughly cleansed (see page 21) is conducted into the water via clear, natural Clear Quartz and indeed strengthened by the Clear Quartz. After 15 minutes, the gem water is ready for use; after two hours it is very intense.

**Advantage:** This is the fastest and most intense of all the preparation methods. As with the test tube method, it is suitable for use with any crystals including toxic, waxed or oiled.

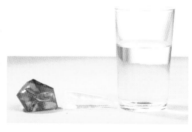

**Disadvantage:** As crystals also radiate energy from their surfaces it passes into the air surrounding the crystal, which is not always desirable; so we recommend that you only use this method in the open air, or somewhere you can be sure that it will not disturb anyone.

If this is not possible, 'shield' the crystals with leather, black silk or a similar material.

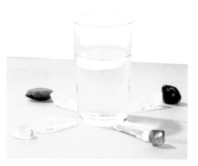

### Glass of water on a crystal slice

First cleanse the crystal slice as described on page 21, then pour the water into a drinking glass and place it on top of the crystal slice. The gem water will be ready to decant after four to 16 hours. Producing the gem water under good hygienic conditions makes a longer period of preparation possible.

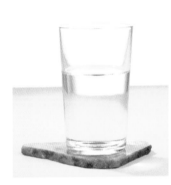

**Advantage:** This method is ideal because it is so simple; also, you can use oiled or waxed crystals to prepare the gem water with this method.

**Disadvantage:** The thickness of the bottom of the glass will slow the absorption of the information. Cheap glass also contains traces of metals, which will release additional information. The range of crystals suitable for use as slices is also limited.

### Water in crystal bowls

With this method, first cleanse a crystal bowl as described on page 21, then pour the water into the bowl. The gem water will be ready to decant after two to eight hours. With this method, you can leave the water for longer periods of preparation and also top up the water to produce the gem water on a continuous basis.

**Advantage:** With this method, you don't need to use a glass container, which may itself convey information. Also, certain types of crystal (such as Jasper, Nebula Stone, etc) protect the water from undesirable influences.

**Disadvantage:** Any wax on waxed crystal bowls needs to be removed beforehand. Also, the range of crystals available in this form is very limited.

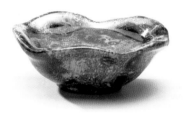

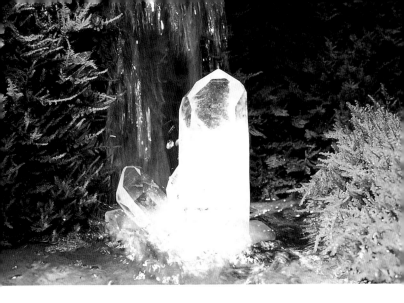

## *Effects and applications*

Gem waters produce intense effects and can be used in a variety of ways, from purifying your living or working space to bathing and taking internally for therapeutic remedies. There are almost as many, if not more, uses as there are crystals themselves, though from the point of view of visual appeal, the crystals simply cannot be beaten.

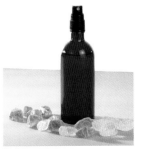

### Using externally

**Cleansing a room:** Place some gem water in a bottle with a spray mechanism and spray it around the rooms in which you live and work to energetically cleanse and improve the atmosphere.

Depending on the crystal used, you can clear relevant room spaces of undesirable influences and at the same time activate the calming properties of the gems.

**Energetic balance:** Spray gem water in the energetic field (aura) surrounding the body to activate its calming or balancing effects on the meridians and chakras and also to strengthen the aura so that it offers better energetic protection.

**Spraying onto the skin:** In the case of wounds, itching, sunburn or skin complaints, it can be more effective to spray gem water onto the affected area than to apply the crystal itself.

**Washing:** Washing with gem water cleanses and strengthens the skin and the subcutaneous tissues and gem water is therefore often used as a skin tonic. Depending on the crystals used, you can also use it to target certain of the body's systems such as the circulation, or to strengthen others such as the metabolism, or to encourage renewal and regeneration.

**As a compress:** Gem waters can be very effective when applied in the form of a compress to treat injuries such as wounds, pulled muscles and bruises, as well as to encourage scar healing, reduce inflammation, clear lymphatic blockages and even relieve muscle tension.

**Added to a bath:** If intense gem waters are prepared and added to the bath water shortly before bathing, they will cleanse and revitalize and help to relax and lift the mood – again, depending on the type of crystals used. Baths to which gem water has been added are a sensual delight; we have devoted a whole section to them in the chapter called 'Gem water mixtures' (page 41).

## Internal application

**Taking internally:** The most common use of gem water is, of course, to take it internally for healing purposes. Depending on the crystals used,

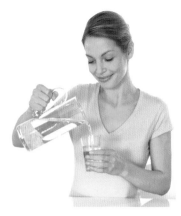

when gem water is taken internally its holistic effects are released on all levels (physical, emotional and spiritual).

**As a mouthwash:** Gargle and rinse your mouth with gem water to treat different complaints, from those affecting the teeth and gums to those affecting the mouth and throat. We have noticed that it can be particularly effective when used to treat inflammation, oral thrush and injuries, as well as after dental treatment.

**For enemas:** Suitable gem waters may also be used to support enemas for cleansing the intestinal tract. They assist in detoxifying and cleansing the gut and in regulating intestinal flora.

You can find information on which gem waters to use for the purposes mentioned above in the chapter called 'Index of crystals for gem water preparation' (page 64), as well as information on how to target the relevant effects. But before you turn to that, please see the following advice on getting the dosage right, which is extremely important.

## Quantity and intensity

Getting the dosage right is the most important factor to consider when gem water is to be taken internally as, once swallowed, the gem water will take its natural course and remain in the body for a certain length of time, acting upon it in some way. It cannot simply be removed again, unlike like a crystal that is worn externally. When gem water is taken internally, it can also act faster and more intensely on the body than healing crystals worn externally.

*It is best to err on the side of caution when taking gem water internally and to begin by taking low doses initially, until you can be sure of the effect it is having and the correct dosage can be determined.*

Use this chart to provide a guide to the amount that can be taken on a daily basis, depending on the effect of the relevant crystal (see the chapter called 'Index of crystals for gem water preparation', page 64):

| Intensity of effect | Initial dose | Maximum dose |
| --- | --- | --- |
| Intensely effective healing crystals | 20 ml (1 shot glass) | 200–500 ml (1–3 drinking glasses) |
| Strongly effective healing crystals | 200–500 ml (1–3 drinking glasses) | 1 litre |
| Gently effective healing crystals | 500 ml–1 litre | unlimited |

As a rule, the daily doses given above can be increased from the initial dose to the maximum dose over the course of a week. For children under fourteen, use half the dose. It goes without saying that you should not treat any illness or psychological problems with gem water without first consulting the doctor or alternative therapist who is treating you or the person you are trying to help.

Exceptions: Although Diamond is classified as an 'intensely effective healing crystal', its maximum dose can still be increased to an unlimited amount (as much as you can drink). With illness such as stroke, you can even begin with a daily dose of 500 ml–1 litre.

Among the 'strongly effective healing crystals' are Apatite, Aquamarine, Fluorite, Moss Agate, Topaz and Tourmaline. The doses for these can also be increased to an unlimited amount. Despite

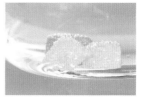

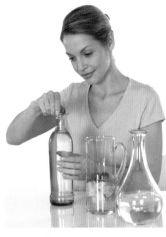

this, care should always be taken with these crystals in all instances.

## Frequency and dosages

In addition to the size of the dose, the frequency with which gem water is taken can also sometimes play an important part. For example, intensely effective gem waters can be better absorbed if they are taken in sips throughout the entire day. By taking many but smaller doses, it is easier to adjust the overall daily dose to an individual's requirements, helping to avoid adverse reactions or taking an excess. In order to take small regulated amounts throughout the day, try putting the whole daily dose in a bottle in the morning and filling up the bottle with suitable water. You can then take the gem water little by little as the day progresses.

**The 'organ clock':** The effect of the gem water will be intensified if you take into account the natural rhythm of the body's different organs.

Each organ – and the functions it performs – reaches a peak of activity at a specific time of day. Taking gem water at the time of the organ's peak activity will ensure the gem water has a much stronger effect on it than taking the same dose at a different time.

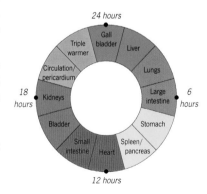

## Initial reactions

The initial 'healing crisis' often experienced in homeopathy (a brief aggravation of symptoms and/or a brief recurrence of some of the symptoms from the past) may also occur with gem waters. This is an indication that the treatment is having some effect, so an initial reaction of this kind can be a reassuring sign that the healing process is beginning. Nevertheless, a healing crisis is occasionally unpleasant and sometimes even violent. If this is the case, it is advisable to stop using the gem water, wait for the reaction to stop, and then to continue using the gem water but at a lower dosage.

## Restrictions for usage

**Physical illness:** In all cases of serious illnesses, especially of the heart and the circulation, nervous complaints, severe infection, as well as any illness that is potentially life-threatening, gem water should only be used after consultation with the doctors and therapists who are treating the patient.

**Mental illness:** In the case of mental illness, gem water should only be used after consulting the doctor or therapist. Mood swings may be triggered by intensely effective gem water, if the sufferer is in a fragile state of mind.

**Pregnancy:** For pregnancy we recommend using gem waters based on crystals that have a more gentle effect. Certain healing crystals, such as Agate, Amber, Chalcedony, Dumortierite, Moonstone, Rose Quartz and Pink Tourmaline (Rubellite) are supportive in pregnancy and may be taken internally as gem water. You should proceed slowly, however, beginning with one to three glasses daily.

Other healing crystals are often better when used externally. You can find out more about using healing crystals during pregnancy in *The Healing Crystal First Aid Manual*, Michael Gienger, Earthdancer, Findhorn Press, 2006.

**Homeopathic therapy:** As having a clear picture of the symptoms being experienced is very important in traditional homeopathy, you should only use gem waters in conjunction with homeopathic treatments after consultation with the homeopathic doctors or therapists treating the problem. If not, the gem water may lead to an incorrect homeopathic diagnosis.

**Counter measures:** If any undesirable or very violent reactions are experienced, they can be alleviated with movement (activity), preferably carried out in the open air, and also by drinking plenty of good water. Saunas, physical activity and sports that cause you to perspire freely will also help the symptoms to disappear faster. The same applies to external contact with water (such as showering or swimming). Taking hot and cold baths alternately, to stimulate the circulation, is the most effective measure. But it is crucial to take into account what your body will tolerate, in terms of its health and constitution; so if you are in the slightest doubt, first consult doctors or therapists that you trust.

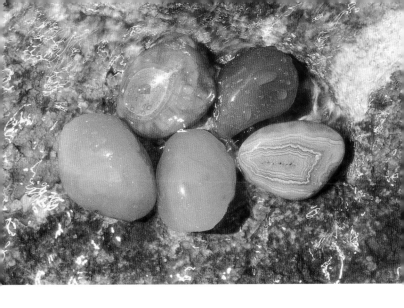

## Gem water mixtures

There is one crucial difference between using crystals in the form of gem water and wearing them or using them externally. If several healing crystals are worn on the body at the same time, the differing kinds of information the crystals convey will often lead to tension. This will sometimes manifest as physical or mental 'conflicts'. The sense of well-being disappears and stress and irritability increase, along with the symptoms of illness. The 'rule of thumb' is to use no more than three different healing crystals at the same time. The rule evolved in 2000, when power bracelets came into fashion, and some wrists were adorned with entire 'garlands of bracelets'.

However, the situation is quite different with gem water. If several crystals are used together in a gem water preparation, the different types of crystal information become integrated during the preparation

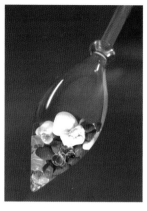

process, creating a new range of information that works differently in combination than it would separately. This is obviously connected with the type of information stored in the water. There are no 'separate memories' but only a 'total memory field'. The conflicts created by the contrary information given by crystals worn externally are partly removed by the harmonizing of information in the gem water. In the case of crystal types that work well together, the different types of information are harmonized – they adapt and balance each other.

## Beware of 'random mixtures'

However, this does not mean that you should prepare gem water mixtures out of healing crystals that are thrown together in a random fashion – the different information they convey could be too different to be harmonized, even by the water. We quite deliberately use the term 'harmonize' rather than 'blend'. Water combines the different types of information into a whole, but whether this new, whole information is 'random' or 'harmonious' still depends on the crystals that are being combined.

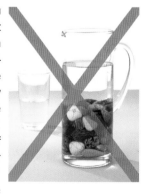

## Important note

Please ensure that you use only those crystals that are suitable for the preparation of gem water (see list of crystals to avoid, pages 13–17). Gem water mixtures should contain five crystals at the very most. Once more, the rule to follow is 'less is more' and in practice we have found that just two or three crystals will normally be sufficient. In order to create gem water mixtures that have a harmonious effect, we also recommend proceeding as follows:

1. **Use your intuition:** Spread out in front of you the crystals that you are intending to use for the preparation and calmly tune into them. What are you feeling? If you feel in harmony with the crystals, you can go ahead and use them as intended. However, if you feel slightly agitated, change the combination by taking away or adding other crystals, until you feel more peaceful and balanced.

2. **Combine related crystals:** In many cases, it has been shown that it is better to combine crystals of the same mineralogical type, rather than to mix those of different types. So quartzes and silicates harmonize very well, as do crystals containing calcium, or those containing magnesium, or copper, or iron. The larger the common mineral content of the crystals, the better they will work together.

But on the other hand, combining those crystals that are recommended for a certain type of healing purpose is no guarantee that the combination will work particularly well. For example, if you were to combine all the crystals that are good for a sore throat in one gem water, it would result in a horrible combination.

3. **Try it out:** As with all good recipes, the same goes for gem water mixtures: 'the proof of the pudding is in the eating'. In other words, you won't really know how well a mixture will work until you try it.

In order to produce a *premier cru* in gem water terms, it is often a case of trial and error. Try a new crystal, or make a small change, and you may soon see better (or worse!) results – but they will all contribute to the learning process.

Here is an example – the objective was to produce a gem water suitable for clearing lymphatic blockages by using Chalcedony, Moss Agate and Opal. A white Precious Opal was initially used. The gem water created proved very successful when used to treat lymph blockages, colds, sensitivity to changes in the weather and many other complaints. However, for reasons of cost, the white Precious Opal was then

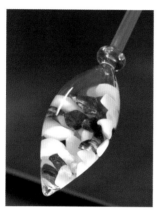

replaced by an ordinary Milky Opal, and the effect remained unchanged. But when the Milky Opal was sometimes replaced by Opalite because of problems with availability, the changes in the effects were quite radical. So why was this? Chalcedony, Moss Agate, Precious Opal and Milky Opal improve the flow of lymph by stimulating the drainage and purification of the lymph. Opalite, on the other hand, supports the purification of the connective tissue, so that toxins and waste products are swept from there into the lymph. However, this could turn out to be problematic if the lymph system is already burdened! So, with the Opalite the detoxification of the tissue is more vigorous; but with Precious Opal and Milky Opal the lymph flow is supported and a self-purification process and cleansing of the lymph channels occurs. Both have their advantages, but they are two completely different processes.

So practical experience is indispensable for creating 'perfected' gem water recipes. In the following pages, we give a number of tried and tested gem water mixtures that we have found to be reliable.

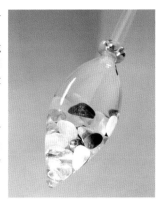

You can follow these 'recipes' yourself, but you can also make your own based on your intuition – you might discover a wonderful new gem water in the process.

### The crystal-clear combination
### Amethyst and Rock Crystal

The combination of these two Quartzes supports mental clarity and bestows alertness, consciousness and good observational abilities, as well as the faculty for mediating and settling conflicts peaceably. On a physical level, the mixture is beneficial for the brain, the nerves, the skin and the intestines, for dissolving respiratory blockages, and for alleviating pain, bruises and swellings. Like the 'basic mixture' below, the 'crystal-clear combination' can be used long-term as a refreshing drinking water. Important: The Clear Quartz for this mixture should be crystal-clear!

**Preparation:** All methods are suitable.

**Category:** A gently effective mixture.

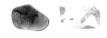

## The basic mixture
### Amethyst, Clear Quartz, Rose Quartz

The so-called 'basic mixture', made out of three quartzes, improves perception, intuition and empathy, has an enlivening and vitalizing effect, encourages inner stability and creates a sense of well-being. Physically, all regulatory mechanisms are harmonized; the brain and nervous system (Amethyst), hormonal system, energy and water balance (Clear Quartz), as well as the circulation and the heart (Rose Quartz). Thus, the mixture supports the balancing of all bodily functions. Note: for long-term use the Rose Quartz should be omitted on a regular basis, as mental alertness will otherwise be impaired.

**Preparation:** All methods are suitable.

**Category:** A gently effective mixture.

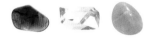

## Setting boundaries and self-determination
### Heliotrope, Nephrite, Serpentine

Boundaries and self-control (Heliotrope), protection and inner peace (Serpentine), as well as strength and inner balance (Nephrite) are combined in a mixture that helps one gain better control of one's own life. A mixture of quartz and silicates for stressful times! Physically, the kidneys, bladder and immune system are strengthened, deacidification is stimulated, inflammations and rheumatic complaints are alleviated, and relaxation and recovery are supported.

**Preparation:** Direct placing in water; the test tube method (especially for 'silver-eye' serpentine, which contains asbestos); conducting with crystals.

**Category:** A gently effective mixture.

## Building strength and regeneration
### Epidote, Nephrite, Ocean Agate, Zoisite

Four green crystals (quartz and silicate) that 'wake one up' and bring 'spring' back into one's life. Recovery (Epidote), constant strength (Nephrite), hope (Ocean Agate) and regeneration (Zoisite) produce a mixture lending high vitality. Very helpful with exhaustion or excessive overtaxing, and to support convalescence following serious illnesses. This mixture is good for the liver, kidneys, triple-warmer and reproductive organs.

**Preparation:** All methods are suitable.

**Category:** A gently effective mixture.

## Liberation and forgiveness
### Mookaite, Obsidian, Rhodonite

A quartz-silicate mixture for resolving conflict and for the healing of physical and psychological traumas. Obsidian dissolves hardening and the retention of old wounds; Rhodonite makes it possible to forgive and to develop new goodwill; Mookaite bestows a positive attitude towards life. In contrast with the emergency mixture, it is suitable for long-term application. Physically, the mixture is useful for improving the blood circulation and quality of the blood, and for wound healing.

**Preparation:** All methods are suitable; however, do not use the boiling method if the Rhodonite contains any black manganese oxide, which may dissolve during boiling.

**Category:** A strongly effective mixture. Start with a low initial dose (see page 37) and increase only very slowly.

## Self-awareness and balance
### Clear Quartz, Red Jasper, Magnesite
Thanks to the contrasting indications of Red Jasper (strength, exertion of all one's energies, activity) and Magnesite (relaxation, letting go and rest), this mixture bestows both vitality and inner composure. Physically, the mixture encourages good blood circulation, warmth and the combustion processes (Jasper), as well as metabolism, digestion and detoxification (Magnesite). It is therefore known as a 'dieting mixture', for which Clear Quartz provides the necessary self-awareness.

**Preparation:** Placing directly in water; test tube method (especially in the case of crumbly Magnesite raw crystals); conducting with crystals.

**Category:** A gently effective mixture.

## Security and trust
### Amazonite, Dumortierite, Rhodonite
Balance, self-determination and trust (Amazonite), ease, confidence and serenity (Dumortierite), as well as understanding, reconciliation and forgiveness (Rhodonite) all contribute to the healing of fears and traumas. This mixture of three silicates helps to overcome powerlessness and the inability to act and to deal with challenges. Works well for travel-sickness, restriction of movement, cramp and pain, as well as disturbances of the autonomic nervous system.

**Preparation:** All methods are suitable; however, do not use the boiling method if the Rhodonite contains any black manganese oxide, which may dissolve during boiling.

**Category:** A strongly effective mixture.

## Harmonious union
### Chrysocolla and Tourmaline

Chrysocolla and Tourmaline are two cyclosilicates, each in its own way encouraging the drive for harmonious union. Chrysocolla encourages balance, aesthetic appreciation and awareness, and a harmonious connection with the environment. Tourmaline (all varieties) encourages inner harmony through a good connection between the spirit, soul, mind and body. Together they create a mixture that can bring order to situations where there is imbalance. Taken internally, the mixture strengthens the brain, the nervous system, the liver, regeneration of tissue and the immune system. Applied externally, it promotes the healing of scars and, with Blue Tourmaline (Indigolite), also of burns.

**Preparation:** Placing crystals directly in water; the test tube method (if some matrix remains on the Chrysocolla; conducting with crystals.

**Category:** A strongly effective mixture.

## Being 'in the flow'
### Chalcedony, Moss Agate, Opal

The quartzes Chalcedony and Moss Agate, as well as Opal (Precious Opal or Milky Opal), which is related to the quartzes, are hydrated silicates; correspondingly they ensure an unhindered, free flow in one's life. Chalcedony enables the free flow of speech and effortless success, while Moss Agate dissolves binding and hampering blocks. Opal makes one flexible, light-hearted and sometimes even a little excessive. Physically this mixture stimulates the lymph flow, which improves the supply of nutrients and waste removal in all the cells and the tissues. The immune system is also strengthened, helping problems ranging from colds and infections through to inflammations with pus. Lymph blockages, joint pains and generally inefficient detoxification are effectively removed.

**Preparation:** All methods are suitable, except for the evaporation and boiling methods, which could damage the Opal.

**Category:** A strongly effective mixture.

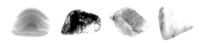

### Clarity of consciousness
### Diamond and Clear Quartz

Used together in gem water, Diamond and Clear Quartz result in a combination that increases the effects of both crystals. The clarity and purity that are characteristics of both crystals are increased to become an invincible striving for spiritual freedom. The mixture helps solve conflicts, problems, uneasy compromises and omissions, until a lasting inner order is established. Discipline, self-observation and clear consciousness are encouraged. In accordance with this, the purification and control of the body are improved, as well as the functioning of the sensory organs, the glands, blood vessels, nerves and the brain. Like the Diamond gem water alone (see page 72), this mixture also provides outstanding help with strokes.

**Preparation:** All methods are suitable.

**Category:** Intensely effective mixture; can be ingested in larger quantities (1 litre/35 fl oz up to an unlimited amount, daily).

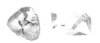

### Strength and flexibility
### Dolomite, Magnesite, Serpentine

The combination of these magnesium minerals in a gem water has a relaxing, calming and stress-alleviating effect. In it are combined balance and contentment (Dolomite) with relaxation, patience and a peaceable nature (Magnesite), as well as protection against pressure and negative external influences (Serpentine).

Physically, the mixture keeps all the muscles relaxed and flexible. It helps with sore muscles, tension and complaints arising from over-exertion, and torn or pulled muscles. It is the ideal choice for sports people – or for breaks, after work, weekends and holidays! It is also excellent for adding to bath water.

**Preparation:** Placing crystals directly in water; the test tube method (with crumbly Dolomite or Magnesite raw crystals, as well as with 'silver-eye' Serpentine containing asbestos); conducting with crystals.

**Category:** A gently effective mixture.

## Purification and clarification
**Amethyst, Diamond, Fluorite, Topaz, Black Tourmaline (Schorl)**

This intense mixture is usually sprayed from a pump-action bottle to clear rooms of negative energies. Amethyst liberates one from attachments; Diamond is intensely clearing, Fluorite dissolves fixed patterns of behaviour, while Tourmaline cleanses and neutralizes, and Topaz provides and protects free spaces. Leave the room immediately after spraying and air it thoroughly for 15 to 30 minutes afterwards, as an intense physical cleansing of the body (diarrhoea, perspiring heavily etc) may also result. If this kind of physical cleansing is desired, then the mixture can be taken internally; however, it is best to do this under the supervision of an expert crystal therapist.

**Preparation:** All methods are suitable.

**Category:** An intensely effective mixture.

## Vitality and truthfulness
### Sodalite and Clear Quartz

The striving for truth and loyalty to oneself (Sodalite) in connection with clarity, awareness and good perception (Clear Quartz) provide a strong mixture in which the individual indications are strengthened. This quartz-silicate mixture helps one to go one's own way but still to be in harmony with the world around. Life flows freely and, correspondingly, water balance in the body is also improved. The kidneys and bladder are strengthened, and water uptake is improved as the mixture stimulates one's natural feeling of thirst. It helps with dry eyes, dry mucous membranes, dry skin or general dehydration and its consequences.

**Preparation:** All methods are suitable.

**Category:** A strongly effective mixture.

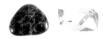

## Happiness and joie de vivre
### Precious Opal, Sunstone, Imperial Topaz

A mixture of three silicates, which helps one's love life! In it, the cheerfulness and love of life of Precious Opal are combined with the confidence and optimism of the Sunstone, as well as the self-confidence of the Imperial Topaz. The mixture removes downheartedness, sorrow and despondency and helps one move through life creatively, with a bounce in one's step. Physically, it improves fertility, and is good for diabetes, metabolic disturbances, digestive problems and nervous disorders.

**Preparation:** All methods are suitable, except the evaporation and boiling method, which might damage the Precious Opal.

**Category:** An intensely effective mixture.

## Study and concentration
### Chrysoberyl, Diamond, Fluorite

An intense mixture for 'lightning perception'. In it, Chrysoberyl encourages concentration, discipline and attentiveness; the Diamond supports stamina, alertness and knowledge, while Fluorite bestows interest, the ability to learn and a rapid grasp of things. The mixture improves one's 'lightning perception' and understanding of unexpected events, along with the systematic learning of large amounts of new material. Physically, it encourages the balancing of the two halves of the brain, coordination, dexterity and the faculty of language. Nerves and sensory organs are strengthened.

**Preparation:** All methods are possible, providing the Chrysoberyl is 100% free of traces of the matrix. Otherwise the test tube method or conducting with crystals is recommended.

**Category:** An intensely effective mixture.

## Pleasure and enjoyment
### Thulite, Mookaite, Rose Quartz

A mixture of silicate and quartzes for the enjoyment of the sensual joys of life; Thulite encourages pleasure and laughter, as well as delight in sexuality, while Mookaite supports the drive for variety and intensely experienced relationships, and Rose Quartz encourages warmth, romance and empathy. Boredom is excluded with this mixture; instead there is enjoyment, fun and sensuality.

Physically, this combination is good for blood formation; it fortifies the circulation and supply with blood, increases fertility and helps with sexual problems.

**Preparation:** All methods are suitable.

**Category:** A strongly effective mixture.

## Openness and wideness
### Apophyllite, Aquamarine and Rutilated Quartz

Liberation and honesty (Apophyllite), directness and farsightedness (Aquamarine), as well as strength of vision and spiritual greatness (Rutilated Quartz) make this combination of silicates and quartz into a mixture that opens up horizons. Narrow-mindedness, faint-heartedness and pedantry disappear and create space for great deeds. Likewise anxieties, worries and feelings of oppression are dispersed. Physically, the mixture helps very well with asthma, allergies and auto-immune reactions.

**Preparation:** Direct placing in water; the test tube method; evaporation method; conducting with crystals.

**Category:** A strongly effective mixture.

  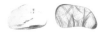

## Maturity and understanding
### Agate, Clear Quartz, Fossil Wood

A quartz mixture for consciousness and mental stability. Agate bestows a sense of security and helps one to become calm; Clear Quartz encourages clear perception and memory; Fossil Wood is grounding and helps one to process experiences. As a mixture they enable one to make sense of and understand life experiences and thus to mature spiritually. Stable integration in one's life and a stable development ensure that nothing will faze one. Physically, this mixture supports the digestion, the metabolism, the connective tissues and the skin, as well as the interaction of the internal organs. Applied externally it is an excellent tonic for stressed skin.

**Preparation:** All methods are suitable.
**Category:** A gently effective mixture.

## Purification and renewal
### Chrysoprase, Ocean Agate, Opalite and Picture Jasper

A quartz-silicate mixture with the effect of a 'spring-cleaning session': Chrysoprase, the most effective detoxification crystal, in combination with the tissue purifiers Opalite and/or Picture Jasper (either of them is sufficient), as well as the Ocean Agate, which generally improves the supply of nutrients and elimination in all the cells and stimulates the lymph flow. This mixture promotes a thorough detoxification and removal of waste products from the body which, interestingly, is more effective, although less violent, than using Chrysoprase alone (see relevant section). This mixture can be used to improve detoxification and even to support cancer treatment (see 'The Healing Crystal First Aid Manual' by Michael Gienger, Earthdancer/Findhorn Press, 2006). On a spiritual level, this mixture cleanses and 'detoxifies', releasing frustration, conflict, sorrow, grief and resentment. Although this may result in moods and mood swings, these can be considered to be signs of healing.

**Preparation:** All methods are suitable.
**Category:** A strongly effective mixture.

## Protection and liberation

**Amethyst, Rock Crystal, Black Tourmaline (Schorl)**

This 'protective' mixture is generally sprayed into the aura (around the body) with a pump-action bottle. The dissolving of attachments (Amethyst), the neutralizing of disturbances (Schorl) and the regaining or maintaining of mental clarity (Clear Quartz) combine to make this quartz-silicate mixture highly effective. It makes one alert and aware and helps to ward off negative influences of any kind, or to process them. In low doses, taken internally, the mixture helps with lazy intestinal activity, diarrhoea and constipation.

**Preparation:** All methods are suitable.

**Category:** An intensely effective mixture.

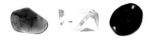

## Alertness of the senses and vitality

**Aquamarine, Clear Quartz, Sardonyx**

Farsightedness (Aquamarine), clarity (Clear Quartz) and sharpened senses (Sardonyx) make this mixture of silicate and quartzes into an elixir for consciousness, perception and insight. At the same time, assiduity, consistency and single-mindedness (Aquamarine), liveliness and a lively, nimble mind (Clear Quartz), as well as virtue and vigour (Sardonyx), bring about the ability to turn insights directly into action. Physically, this mixture gives corresponding strength and stamina, as well as good blood circulation and regeneration and strengthening the kidneys and the bladder. All the sensory organs are supported in their functions.

**Preparation:** All methods are suitable.

**Category:** A strongly effective mixture.

## Sensuality and beauty
### Chrysocolla, Malachite, Turquoise

This is a special mixture for the feminine side in both men and women; the combination of three copper mineral crystals support a sense of beauty, harmony, receptivity and balance: Chrysocolla (copper silicate) encourages caring, 'nurturing' and the physical and spiritual support of others; Malachite (copper carbonate) awakens powers of seduction, sensuality, curiosity and talent for the fine arts; Turquoise (copper aluminium phosphate) represents protecting, caring and self-determination. Physically, the mixture encourages the brain function, sensory perception, detoxification and regeneration. It strengthens the liver, reduces inflammations, kills pain and eases cramp, especially for menstrual complaints.

**Preparation:** Placing crystals directly in water (only crystals with no matrix adhering to them, and only for a maximum of two to four hours in cold water); the test tube method; conducting with crystals.

**Category:** An intensely effective mixture.

## Stability and strengthening
### Coloured Calcites

Calcite is beneficial for the intestine, as it positively influences the intestinal flora and intestinal activity. Calcite gem waters are thus very good for a lazy intestine, constipation, diarrhoea and flatulence. They prevent auto-toxification through decomposition and fermentation processes. As a gem water, the mixture of coloured Calcites has been tried and tested, and the colours appear to bestow additional effects: green has a detoxifying effect; yellow strengthens the digestion; blue regulates water balance; red encourages blood circulation and brown improves elimination. A cleansed intestine also leads to spiritual perception of purity, lightness, strength and liveliness. In addition, the Calcite mixture encourages inner strength and stability, as well as strong development on all levels.

**Preparation:** All methods are suitable.

**Category:** A gently effective mixture.

**A carefree disposition and patience**
**Aventurine and Prase/Prase Quartz**

A combination of green quartzes for free self-determination, good self-control, a quiet disposition and a simple, stress-free life. Aventurine brings relaxation, recovery, regeneration and good sleep, while Prase encourages gentleness, serenity and a good balance between control and release. In this combination the result is self-sufficiency, good-naturedness and contentment. Physically, the mixture works as a painkiller, lowers a temperature, alleviates inflammations and helps with skin complaints (including psoriasis), itching, sunburn and sunstroke, as well as minor burns. For those physical indications it can be used externally and internally.

**Preparation:** All methods are suitable.

**Category:** A gently effective method.

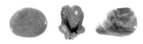

**Growth and development**
**Apatite, Aragonite, Calcite, Fluorite (optional)**

The combination of these calcium minerals has a growth enhancing and regulating effect. Apatite (calcium phosphate) bestows energy, stimulates growth and strengthens cartilage and bone. Aragonite (rhombic calcium carbonate) regulates growth, especially in processes that are proceeding too fast. Calcite (trigonal calcium carbonate) strengthens growth through a healthy metabolism and brings stability on all levels. Together, the three provide a 'growth mixture' for children as well as for adults with problems with bones and joints. The mixture also works well on a spiritual level: Apatite stimulates spiritual development, Aragonite balances it and Calcite stabilizes it. If Fluorite (calcium fluoride) is added, any developments (physical, emotional, spiritual, mental) that have gone wrong are corrected or 'put back in order' again. With Fluorite the mixture will also help with cases of ganglions, or joints that have become stiff. Order and flexibility are correspondingly also the spiritual themes of Fluorite.

**Preparation:** All methods except the boiling method are suitable.

**Category:** A gently effective mixture.

## The emergency gem water
### Obsidian, Rhodonite, Amethyst, Clear Quartz

This mixture of silicates and quartzes provides intense, fast-working support for shocks and injuries, as well as traumatic experiences of a physical or emotional nature. Obsidian is the shock releaser, which has a pain-alleviating effect. Rhodonite is the number 1 wound-healing crystal for physical and emotional traumas and also helps overcome anxieties and panic. Amethyst helps one overcome spiritual confusion and also contributes towards overcoming sadness and emotional states. Finally, Clear Quartz makes one clear and aware, helps one see things as they are, and thus encourages the immediate mental processing of things one has experienced. The mixture can be taken internally as well as being sprayed around the body or directly on the injured parts of the body. It very quickly leads to clarity of the mind and the alleviation of pain; it also greatly improves the healing of wounds.

**Preparation:** All methods are suitable, however, the boiling method should only be used if the Rhodonite does not contain any manganese oxide, which might possibly be dissolved during boiling.

**Category:** An intensely effective mixture.

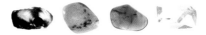

### The five-element mixture

Ocean Agate, Rose Quartz, Fossil Wood, Amethyst, Chalcedony

This mixture consists of five quartzes which, within the combination, each individually represent one element according to Chinese medicine. Traditional Chinese medicine (TCM) sees good health as the ability to change, that is, the ability to deal with changed circumstances or situations. We only become ill if we are no longer able to change, and a complete standstill means death. Every change in life, no matter how small or large, passes through five stages: the wood phase 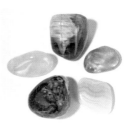 (Phase of Beginning), the fire phase (Phase of Expansion), the earth phase (Phase of Balance), the metal phase (Phase of Contraction) and the water phase (Phase of Ending). Changes proceed harmoniously if there are no disturbances in any of the phases. Thus the crystals of the 'five-element mixture' were chosen so that, on the one hand, they can eliminate the disturbances in the five phases of change, and on the other hand, will harmonize well with each other. The following mixture has turned out to be an optimal one.

- **Phase of Change – Wood:** Ocean Agate as a crystal for the 'principle of hope', for renewal, building up and regeneration.

- **Phase of Change – Fire:** Rose Quartz as the crystal for love, warmth, joie de vivre, sensuality and sexuality.
- **Phase of Change – Earth:** Fossil Wood as a crystal for balance, changeable stability and deep rooting.
- **Phase of Change – Metal:** Amethyst as the crystal for inner peace and meditation, as well as for alertness and awareness.
- **Phase of Change – Water:** Blue Chalcedony as the crystal for inner flexibility and a constant flow of vitality.

This mixture keeps one full of vitality and health, leads to a beneficial balance of activity and relaxation and promotes a positive attitude towards life. This makes it an 'all round mixture' that will have a supportive effect in all situations of life. In addition, the five-element mixture can be used diagnostically with the help of the sense of taste: there is a typical taste for every phase of change, which can be used as an indicator when drinking the mixture, and tells us which element we need most at that moment.

- If we need wood, the water tastes sour.
- If we need fire, the water tastes bitter.
- If we need earth, the water tastes sweet.
- If we need metal, the water tastes sharp or metallic.
- If we need water, the water tastes (slightly) salty.

This effect was not planned or intended, but showed up quite unexpectedly during the first tests with the mixture. However, as these sensitive perceptions of taste exactly correspond with the teachings of TCM, and appear to correspond with the symptoms displayed by the person in question, this result is a clear confirmation that the mixture does indeed represent all the five elements and brings about a balance.

**Preparation:** All methods are suitable.

**Category:** A gently effective mixture.

## Gem water bath additives

Gem water can also be used as a bath additive. For this purpose, the preparation process needs to be as long as possible, in order to create a very intense gem water. Use the maximum length indicated in the chapter 'Effects and Applications' for one litre of water and carry out the preparation of the gem water for 12 to 24 hours (with direct placing in water), or four to six hours, if conducting with crystals. Add the gem water to the bath water shortly before stepping into the bath. Depending on the types of crystals, you can prepare various different kinds of baths:

**A relaxing bath:** Aventurine, Magnesite, Prase, Serpentine, Turquoise

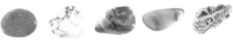

**A stress-relieving bath:** Chrysocolla, Dumortierite, Smoky Quartz, Black Tourmaline (Schorl)

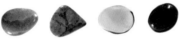

**A stimulating bath:** Amber, Calcite, Orange Citrine, Sunstone, Imperial Topaz

**A revitalizing bath:** Epidote, Red Garnet, Heliotrope, Carnelian, Mookaite, Zoisite

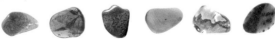

**A bath for the skin:** Agate, Amethyst, Clear Quartz, Dumortierite, Fluorite, Rose Quartz

**A purifying bath:** Amazonite, Blue Chalcedony, Chrysoprase, Kambaba Jasper, Moss Agate, Nephrite, Ocean Agate (Ocean Jasper), Emerald

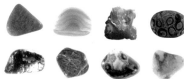

**A sensual bath:** Fire Opal, Red Garnet, Rhodochrosite, Rose Quartz, Thulite, Red Tourmaline (Rubellite)

The crystals listed do not represent a fixed mixture, but rather a selection for you to combine following your own intuition – without any claims to being complete. Please make your own choices, and do not use all the crystals listed all at once! One to three crystals will suffice as a rule. Intuitively choose those that appeal to you most.

Do not place the crystals directly in the bath water, but prepare the gem water as described above. Their effectiveness will thus be much greater, and the crystals will not be damaged in any way. The latter is particularly important if you are also using essential oils or other bath additives. The warm water and the substances dissolved in the bath water are not good for some crystals. However, you will be able to create a wonderful sense of well-being with the gem waters and other bath additives.

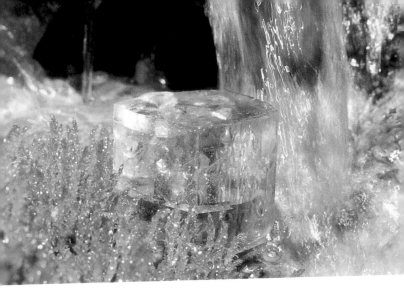

## Index of crystals for gem water preparation

The following index presents the mineralogical features of the crystals in common use for gem water preparation, together with a description of their healing properties. Please note that not all the known healing effects of the crystals in the list are included in the descriptions, as these have already been documented in previous books and would exceed the scope of this little handbook*. Instead, the emphasis here is on the effects associated with gem waters in particular.

* See also, Michael Gienger, *Crystal Power, Crystal Healing (The Complete Handbook)*, Blandford, 1998; Michael Gienger, *Healing Crystals: A–Z to 430 Gemstones*, Earthdancer/ Findhorn Press, 2005; *The Healing Crystal First Aid Manual*, Earthdancer/Findhorn Press, 2006.

You will find the following information in detail in this index:

**Title:** The heading of each entry gives the name of the featured crystal. In addition to the mineralogical name, we give the trade name(s) if it helps to identify the crystal or describe it. To make a distinction between the two, the scientific names are in black and trade names in blue.

**Mineralogy:** This gives a brief description of the mineral class and, if appropriate, the mineral group, as well as the crystal system and the way it was formed ('primary' = magmatic formation, 'secondary' = through weathering and sedimentation, 'tertiary' = metamorphic formation under pressure and heat). In addition to the crystal colour, these are very important in relation to its healing effect and application.

**Indications:** Here we list the most significant healing effects or the particular area of effectiveness of each crystal used to prepare gem waters. We also highlight any additional aspects that came to light when using the gem water.

**Preparation:** This section defines the appropriate methods of preparation for each crystal. Placing the crystal directly in water, the boiling method and the evaporation method should only be used for crystals that are specifically suitable – otherwise you risk damaging the crystals or, even worse, damaging your health. The test tube method is suitable for all crystals, but is only indicated if we recommend that you avoid placing a particular crystal directly in the water.

**Category:** The final section defines the effect of each crystal as gentle, strong or intense. These categories will help you decide on the correct number of crystals to use in the preparation of gem waters (see page 27), as well as the right dosage for taking internally (see page 37), so please use the information to help you get the best result.

---

**Abbreviations used pages 67–91:** trig. = trigonal, monocl. = monoclinic, orthorh. = orthorhombic, hex. = hexagonal, am. = amorphous, prim. = primary, sec. = secondary, tert. = tertiary

## Agate

**Mineralogy:** Banded Quartz (silicon dioxide, trigonal, primary)

**Indications:** Protection, stability, security, spiritual serenity, maturity. For the eyes, hollow organs (stomach, intestine, bladder, womb, etc), blood vessels, connective tissues, skin and mucous membranes. Encourages digestion, elimination, growth and regeneration. Protective crystal for pregnancy.

**Preparation:** All methods are suitable.

**Category:** A gently effective gem water.

## Amazonite (Feldspar)

**Mineralogy:** Potassium feldspar (tectosilicate, triclinic, prim./tert.)

**Indications:** Self-determination, responsibility for self, balance, inner harmony, trust. Alleviates heart problems caused by grief. For the metabolism, the liver, tendons, joints, brain, autonomic nervous system, pituitary gland and thymus gland. Relaxing and for alleviating cramp (also while giving birth).

**Preparation:** All methods are suitable.

**Category:** A strongly effective gem water.

## Amber

**Mineralogy:** Fossilized tree resin (organic, amorphous, secondary)

**Indications:** Self-awareness, carefreeness, happiness, cheerfulness. Good for the liver, gall bladder, stomach, intestines, pancreas, spleen, nerves, thyroid gland, metabolism, digestion, detoxification, elimination, skin, mucous membranes and joints. Helps with allergies, diabetes, nausea, pain in the limbs, rheumatism and gout.

**Preparation:** All methods are suitable except the boiling method.

**Category:** A gently effective gem water.

## Amethyst

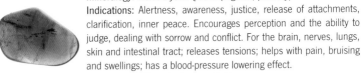

**Mineralogy:** Violet crystal Quartz (trigonal, primary)

**Indications:** Alertness, awareness, justice, release of attachments, clarification, inner peace. Encourages perception and the ability to judge, dealing with sorrow and conflict. For the brain, nerves, lungs, skin and intestinal tract; releases tensions; helps with pain, bruising and swellings; has a blood-pressure lowering effect.

**Preparation:** All methods are suitable.

**Category:** A gently effective gem water.

## Ametrine

**Mineralogy:** Yellow-violet crystal Quartz (trigonal, primary)

**Indications:** Cheerful serenity, fulfilled existence, joie de vivre, optimism, well-being, inner balance. Helps meet great demands with inner composure. Harmonizes the two halves of the brain, the autonomic nervous system and the metabolism; brings a balanced natural tension in the body.

**Preparation:** All methods are suitable.

**Category:** A gently effective gem water.

## Antimonite

**Mineralogy:** Dark grey antimony sulphide (orthorhombic, primary)

**Indications:** Positive attitude towards life; creative power; harmonizing of personal interests with higher ideals. Helps change an aversion to mortal existence into a life filled with meaning. For complaints with the digestion (stomach), the gums and the skin (psoriasis). In conjunction with sulphur elixir, good for psoriasis (apply externally!).

**Preparation:** Test tube method, conducting with crystals.

**Category:** A strongly effective gem water.

## Apatite

**Mineralogy:** Calcium phosphate (hexagonal, primary/tertiary)

**Indications:** Openness, enjoying contacts, liveliness, drive, motivation. Lends energy to support great effort and exhaustion; encourages a healthy appetite. For growth, teeth and bones; helps with osteoporosis, bone fractures, osteoarthritis and joint complaints.

**Preparation:** Direct placing in water; test tube method (with crumbly raw crystals); conducting with crystals.

**Category:** Strongly effective; possible to take large amounts.

## Apophyllite

**Mineralogy:** Hydrated phyllosilicate (tetragonal, primary)

**Indications:** Composure, calmness, honesty, straightforwardness, openness, liberation. Releases feelings of oppression, uncertainty, worries and anxieties; liberates from retained feelings. Helps with complaints of the nerves, skin, bladder and mucous membranes; respiratory problems (sore throat, bronchitis); allergies and asthma.

**Preparation:** Direct placing in water; conducting with crystals.

**Category:** A strongly effective gem water.

### Aquamarine

**Mineralogy:** Beryl containing iron, blue to green (hexagonal, primary)
**Indications:** Spiritual growth, farsightedness, serenity, discipline, concentration. Makes one honest, focused, dynamic, full of stamina and successful. Helps with allergies (hay fever!), autoimmune diseases, hyperactivity, eye complaints, throat and stomach pains, nausea, kidney, bladder and thyroid gland problems.
**Preparation:** All methods are suitable.
**Category:** A strongly effective gem water.

### Aragonite

**Mineralogy:** Calcium carbonate (orthorhombic, secondary)
**Indications:** Regulation of growth processes; balancing in cases of too rapid development. Unburdening when overly great demands are made on one; inner restlessness and nervousness. For calcium metabolism, muscles, bones, spinal discs, meniscus, digestion, stomach and intestines. 'Onyx marble' (Aragonite-Calcite) can also be used for this.
**Preparation:** All methods are suitable except for the boiling method.
**Category:** A gently effective gem water.

### Aventurine, green

**Mineralogy:** Glittering Quartz containing Fuchsite (trigonal, primary)
**Indications:** A carefree attitude, relaxation, peace of the soul; acceptance of life's circumstances. Aids recovery, regeneration and healthy sleep. Preventive for arteriosclerosis and heart attack; helps with nervousness, stress and pain; alleviates skin eruptions, itching, allergies, inflammations, sunburn and sunstroke.
**Preparation:** All methods are suitable.
**Category:** A gently effective gem water.

### Azurite

**Mineralogy:** Basal copper carbonate (monoclinic, secondary)
**Indications:** A drive for experience and insight; dissolving of programming from the past. Encourages awareness; makes one thoughtful, critical and fast to react. Stimulates the brain and nervous activities; stimulates the thyroid gland and growth; alleviates pain; eases cramp; detoxifies and stimulates the liver.
**Preparation:** Test tube method; conducting with crystals.
**Category:** An intensely effective gem water.

## Bronzite

**Mineralogy:** Inosilicate of the pyroxene group (orthorhombic, prim.)

**Indications:** Composure and drive. For dealing with life when great demands are made. Brings strength from inner peace, as well as recovery through even the shortest period of rest. Helps with stress; strengthens the nerves; eases cramp and alleviates pain. In combination with Apatite it encourages the stability and hardness of bones.

**Preparation:** All methods are suitable.

**Category:** A strongly effective gem water.

## Calcite

**Mineralogy:** Calcium carbonate (trigonal, secondary)

**Indications:** Stability, self-confidence, steadfastness, healthy growth, harmonious development. Combats laziness; strengthens the ability to surmount difficulties; makes one capable and successful. Regulates the metabolism, digestion and elimination. Good for bones, teeth, connective tissues, the skin, mucous membranes and the intestines.

**Preparation:** All methods are suitable except the boiling method.

**Category:** A gently effective gem water.

## Carnelian

**Mineralogy:** Chalcedony containing Hematite (quartz, trigonal, prim.)

**Indications:** Courage, overcoming difficulties, willingness to help, sociability, pragmatism, removing inhibitions. Stabilizes circulation and supply with blood; helps with very low blood pressure; staunches blood; improves blood quality; stimulates the small intestine and metabolism. Helps rheumatic complaints and brings out fevers if necessary.

**Preparation:** All methods are suitable.

**Category:** A strongly effective gem water.

## Celestite (Celestine)

**Mineralogy:** Strontium sulphate (orthorhombic, sec./rarely primary)

**Indications:** Relief, strengthening and stability. Dissolves feelings of heaviness, constriction, oppression and powerlessness. Brings structure into one's life, thinking and work. Helps with lack of strength and exhaustion; relieves chronic muscle tension, as well as hardening in the bones, tissues and organs.

**Preparation:** Test tube method; conducting with crystals.

**Category:** A gently effective gem water.

## Chalcedony, blue

**Mineralogy:** Fibrous quartz (trigonal, primary/secondary)
**Indications:** Communication, understanding, ease, being in the flow. Lowers blood pressure and high temperatures; encourages lactation and lymph flow. Good for the respiratory organs, mucous membranes, thyroid gland, kidneys, bladder, and sensitivity to changes in weather; helps with pains in the limbs, inflammations, allergies and diabetes.
**Preparation:** All methods are suitable.
**Category:** A gently effective gem water.

## Chalcedony, pink (Rose Chalcedony)

**Mineralogy:** Chalcedony containing manganese (Quartz, trig., sec.)
**Indications:** Warm-heartedness, liveliness, trust, goodness and help-fulness. Encourages openness, the ability to listen and understand, and clear heart-to-heart communication. Encourages lactation in nursing mothers; helps with diabetes, weak immune response and colds, as well as heart disease resulting from chronic infection.
**Preparation:** All methods are suitable.
**Category:** A gently effective gem water.

## Charoite

**Mineralogy:** Phyllo or sheet silicate rich in minerals (monocl., tert.)
**Indications:** Determination, spontaneity, drive. Lends composure in stressful situations; helps to overcome compulsions and resistance, make important decisions, and deal with mountains of work. Calms the nerves, induces restful sleep, helps alleviate pain, eases cramp and helps with disturbances of the autonomic nervous system.
**Preparation:** Test tube method; conducting with crystals.
**Category:** An intensely effective gem water.

## Chiastolite

**Mineralogy:** Aluminium silicate with carbon inclusions (orthorh., tert.)
**Indications:** Identity, sobriety, alertness, a sense of reality, identifying one's soul purpose or life's task. Helps with nervousness, anxieties and feelings of guilt. Alleviates over-acidification, rheumatism and gout, strengthens the nerves, helps with exhaustion, states of physical weakness, impaired perception and movement, as well as with paralysis.
**Preparation:** All methods are suitable.
**Category:** A strongly effective gem water.

## Chrysoberyl

**Mineralogy:** Aluminium beryl oxide (orthorhombic, primary/tertiary)
**Indications:** Self-control, discipline, strictness, authority, control. Helps with anxieties, feelings of oppression, stress, nervousness and hyperactivity; encourages concentration, ability to learn and strategic thinking. Balances the two halves of the brain; helps with speech impediments and sensory disorders. Strengthens the liver.
**Preparation:** All methods are suitable.
**Category:** An intensely effective gem water.

## Chrysocolla

**Mineralogy:** Hydrated copper silicate (monoclinic, secondary)
**Indications:** Balance, caring, harmony. For keeping a cool head under stress, nervousness, irritability, mood swings and strong emotions. Strengthens the liver and brain; cools, relaxes, detoxifies and lowers high blood pressure. For infections, throat inflammations, fevers, pain, scars, cramp, menstrual complaints.
**Preparation:** Test tube method; conducting with crystals.
**Category:** A strongly effective gem water.

## Chrysoprase

**Mineralogy:** Chalcedony containing nickel (quartz, trigonal, sec.)
**Indications:** Security, trust, resolution of conflicts, patience. For jealousy, lovesickness, problems in relationships, nightmares, burdens, sexual problems. For detoxification and elimination; strengthens the liver, gall bladder, kidneys, intestines. For allergies, rheumatism, gout, skin diseases, fungal infections, herpes, neurodermatitis, psoriasis.
**Preparation:** All methods, as long as no matrix is attached.
**Category:** An intensely effective gem water.

## Citrine

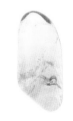

**Mineralogy:** Yellow crystalline quartz (silicon dioxide, trigonal, prim.)
**Indications:** Self-expression, self-confidence, courage for life, joie de vivre. For dynamism and variety; improves processing of experiences. Helps with grief, depression, bed-wetting and growth disorders. Has a warming effect; strengthens the nerves, digestion, stomach, spleen and pancreas, so good for diabetes.
**Preparation:** All methods are suitable.
**Category:** Strongly effective; possible to take large amounts.

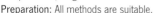

## Clear Quartz

**Mineralogy:** Clear Quartz (trigonal, primary)

**Indications:** Clarity, awareness, neutrality, a firm standpoint. Strengthens perception, attentiveness, memory and understanding. A good distributor of energy; lowers high temperatures; alleviates pain. Harmonizes brain, nerves, glands and hormonal and water balance. Good for the skin, hair and nails. Increases the effects of other crystals.

**Preparation:** All methods are suitable.

**Category:** A gently effective gem water.

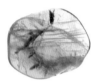

## Cordierite (Iolite; Dichroite)

**Mineralogy:** Magnesium aluminium cyclosilicate (orthorhombic, tert.)

**Indications:** Unshakeability, self-confidence, stamina, patience, staying power. Helps to bear the most adverse circumstances, to take on responsibility and to carry out duties. Improves efficiency; strengthens the nerves; helps with paralysis and numbness in the limbs; alleviates pain and nervous bladder complaints.

**Preparation:** All methods are suitable.

**Category:** A strongly effective gem water.

## Diamond

**Mineralogy:** Pure carbon (natural elements, cubic, tertiary)

**Indications:** Invincibility, control, liberation from compulsions, virtue, insight, honesty, strong character, self-determination, spiritual freedom. Helps with anxiety and depression. Encourages purification and control over one's life; supports the sensory organs, hormone glands, blood vessels, nerves and the brain. The best healing aid after strokes!

**Preparation:** Direct placing in water; conducting with crystals.

**Category:** Intensely effective; possible to take large amounts.

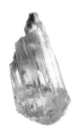

## Diaspore

**Mineralogy:** Aluminium oxide hydroxide (orthorhombic, tertiary)

**Indications:** Finding one's own identity; revival of original goals; perceiving and changing relationship structures. Stimulates self-analysis and making corrections to one's life. Encourages the digestion; helps with heartburn and stomach complaints; the best gem water for excess acid.

**Preparation:** Direct placing in water; conducting with crystals.

**Category:** A gently effective gem water.

## Diopside

**Mineralogy:** Inosilicate of the pyroxene group (monoclinic, tertiary)

**Indications:** Forgiving, letting go, reconciliation. Dissolving of old pain and injuries; helps to make peace. Brings vitality; strengthens the kidneys; improves the balance of hormones, acid/base, minerals and water in the body. Harmonizes muscle tone and vascular tension; improves nerve reactions.

**Preparation:** All methods are suitable.

**Category:** A gently effective gem water.

## Dioptase

**Mineralogy:** Hydrated copper silicate (trigonal, secondary)

**Indications:** Wealth, beauty, good fortune. Brings hope, depth of feeling, a multitude of ideas, intense dreams and creativity. Helps place one in the right light. Accelerates healing processes; strengthens the liver, spinal discs, meniscus and eyes; encourages regeneration; alleviates pain, cramp and chronic headaches.

**Preparation:** Test tube method; conducting with crystals.

**Category:** An intensely effective gem water.

## Disthene, blue (Cyanite, Kyanite)

**Mineralogy:** Aluminium silicate (triclinic, tertiary)

**Indications:** Preserving one's own identity; completing one's soul purpose or life's task. Encourages logical-rational thinking, self-control and accomplishing tasks. Helps to bear pain, and to remain able to act in extreme situations. Alleviates hoarseness and complaints affecting the larynx; good for body control, motor activity and dexterity.

**Preparation:** All methods are suitable.

**Category:** A strongly effective gem water.

## Dolomite

**Mineralogy:** Calcium magnesium carbonate (trigonal, secondary)

**Indications:** Self-discovery, talents, sense of community, patience, balance, contentment. Relaxes; helps gain and maintain vitality. Eases cramp; alleviates pain, waste deposits in blood vessels and a tendency to thrombosis. Good for blood, blood vessels, heart, circulation and complaints caused by metabolic imbalance.

**Preparation:** All methods are suitable except the boiling method.

**Category:** A gently effective gem water.

## Dumortierite

**Mineralogy:** Aluminium boro-silicate (orthorhombic, primary)

**Indications:** Carefreeness, serenity, courage, faith, trust. Helps with nervousness, stress, compulsion, panic, anxieties, homesickness, grief and depression. For the intestines, skin, gall bladder; for travel-sickness, nausea, vomiting, diarrhoea, colic, headaches, nervous complaints, epilepsy and sensory imbalances.

**Preparation:** All methods are suitable.

**Category:** A gently effective gem water.

## Emerald

**Mineralogy:** Beryl containing chromium (cyclosilicate, hex., prim./tert.)

**Indications:** Direction; growth; finding a purpose in things; harmony; unity with partners. Strengthens the immune system; helps with infections and inflammations. Good for the eyes, respiratory tract, heart, liver, gall bladder and intestine. Has a detoxifying effect; helps with rheumatism, gout, pain, cramp, headache, neurodermatitis and epilepsy.

**Preparation:** All methods, as long as no matrix is attached.

**Category:** An intensely effective gem water.

## Epidote-Feldspar (Unakite)

**Mineralogy:** Epidote-Feldspar compound (monoclinic, prim./tert.)

**Indications:** Recovery, regeneration, regaining health after an illness. Good after serious illnesses or great exhaustion. Helps with overwork, self-pity, grief, sorrow and frustration. Improves efficiency, the constitution and physical condition; fortifies the liver, gall bladder, digestion and the immune system. Accelerates the healing processes.

**Preparation:** All methods are suitable.

**Category:** A gently effective gem water.

## Falcon's Eye (Hawk's Eye, blue Tiger's Eye)

**Mineralogy:** Quartz with Crocidolite inclusions (trigonal, primary)

**Indications:** Overview, distance, powers of observation. Alleviates pain, helps with nervousness, inner unrest, trembling and excess hormonal functioning. Makes it possible to preserve an overview in complicated situations and helps with making difficult decisions.

**Preparation:** Direct placing into water; the test tube method (for fibrous raw crystals); conducting with crystals.

**Category:** A gently effective gem water.

## Fire Opal

**Mineralogy:** Red to yellow Precious Opal containing iron (am., prim.)
**Indications:** Lust for life, enjoyment, enthusiasm, a wealth of ideas, spontaneity, cheerfulness, eroticism, joy of sexuality. Makes one wide awake, fast and efficient; helps with tiredness, weakness and low blood pressure; encourages blood circulation, potency and fertility.
**Preparation:** Direct placing into water (only crystals without attached matrix); test tube method; conducting with crystals.
**Category:** An intensely effective gem water.

## Fluorite

**Mineralogy:** Calcium fluoride (halide, isometric, mostly primary)
**Indications:** Order, self-determination, flexibility, interest, free spirit. Encourages concentration, thinking and learning; promotes clarity. Regulates growth; strengthens teeth and bones; helps with ganglions and joint problems. Good for the skin, mucous membranes, respiratory system, lungs, intestines, nerves and brain. Alleviates allergies.
**Preparation:** All methods (do not place Antozonite directly in water)
**Category:** Strongly effective; possible to take large amounts.

## Fossil Wood

**Mineralogy:** Wood transformed into Quartz (trigonal, secondary)
**Indications:** Grounding, stability, deep rooting; the ability to change. Bestows down-to-earthness, contentment, recovery, well-being and a good body image. Beneficial for homesickness. Effective for calming the nerves, for the digestion, metabolism and elimination, as well as against overweight caused by 'lack of grounding'.
**Preparation:** All methods are suitable.
**Category:** A gently effective gem water.

## Garnet, red

**Mineralogy:** Red aluminium nesosilicate (cubic, tertiary)
**Indications:** Willpower, the strength to resist, strong will, courage, hope, good quality of life, helpfulness in crises; for tiredness, weakness and exhaustion. Encourages sexuality, potency, muscular strength, the metabolism, the circulation and the quality of the blood. Strengthens the immune system.
**Preparation:** All methods are suitable except the boiling method.
**Category:** An intensely effective gem water.

## Grossular Garnet

**Mineralogy:** Calcium aluminium nesosilicate (cubic, tertiary)

**Indications:** Building up, strengthening, regeneration, orientation, reordering. Bestows new perspectives, hope; willingness to give and receive help. Strengthens the liver and kidneys; alleviates inflammations; helps with gall bladder problems, rheumatism and arthritis; detoxifies and regenerates the skin and mucous membranes.

**Preparation:** All methods are suitable except the boiling method.

**Category:** A strongly effective gem water.

## Halite (Salt Stone, Salt Crystal)

**Mineralogy:** Sodium chloride (halide, cubic, secondary)

**Indications:** Protection, purification, inner balance. Dissolves patterns of unconscious thinking and behaviour; helps with subtle energetic influences. Regulates the metabolism and water balance in the body; detoxifies; eliminates waste products; good for the respiratory system, the intestines and the skin.

**Preparation:** Test tube method; conducting with crystals.

**Category:** A strongly effective gem water.

## Heliotrope

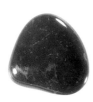

**Mineralogy:** Green Jasper with red flecks (trigonal, secondary)

**Indications:** Protection, shielding, boundaries. Improves control over one's own life. Strengthens the immune system; helps with infections, influenza, colds, inflammations, formation of pus. For the heart, eyes, ears, respiratory organs, intestines, liver, gall bladder, bladder, lymph system and blood vessels. A good preventive against heart attacks.

**Preparation:** All methods are suitable.

**Category:** A gently effective gem water.

## Hematite

**Mineralogy:** Iron oxide (trigonal, primary/tertiary)

**Indications:** Vitality, liveliness, the strength for survival, commitment, progress. Supports the improvement of life's circumstances and the realization of one's own goals. Improves the absorption of iron, formation of blood and the supply of oxygen to all the cells and organs.

**Preparation:** All methods are suitable; test tube method preferable, or conducting with crystals (no release of iron into the water).

**Category:** A gently effective gem water.

## Jadeite (Jade)

**Mineralogy:** Inosilicate of the pyroxene group (monoclinic, tertiary)

**Indications:** Balance, inner balance, self-realization. Creates a balance between rest and activity; enlivens dreams and visualizations and helps to renew energy reserves. Regulates the nerves, the kidneys and adrenals (adrenalin production); helps with the balance of water, mineral substances and acid/bases in the body.

**Preparation:** All methods are suitable.

**Category:** A gently effective gem water.

## Jasper, red

**Mineralogy:** Jasper containing Hematite (quartz, trigonal, secondary)

**Indications:** Willpower, courage, readiness for conflict, honesty, strength, steadfastness. Makes one lively, dynamic, courageous, mentally active, straightforward and direct. Brings energy; helps to put ideas into action. Regulates temperature, circulation and supply with blood. Lowers temperatures; helps with weakness and tiredness.

**Preparation:** All methods are suitable.

**Category:** A strongly effective gem water.

## Jet (Gagate)

**Mineralogy:** Carbon rock rich in bitumen (amorphous, secondary)

**Indications:** Optimism, tenacity, steadfastness, unshakeability, dignity. Helps overcome sorrow, grief, pessimism and depression; helps one to accept that which cannot be changed, but steadfastly to change what can be changed. Helps with complaints with the mouth, gums, intestines (diarrhoea), the skin, joints and the spine.

**Preparation:** Test tube method; conducting with crystals.

**Category:** A gently effective gem water.

## Kabamba stone (Rhyolite)

**Mineralogy:** Quartz Anorthoclase Riebeckite Aegirine vulcanite (prim.)

**Indications:** Vitality; ability to cope with burdens; level-headedness, wish fulfilment, protection. Helps with anxieties, doubts and worries. Stimulates bodily fluids; regulates perspiration; detoxifies; eliminates waste products; fortifies the immune system. Good for influenza, colds and inflammations of the lungs, intestines, stomach, kidneys, bladder.

**Preparation:** All methods except the boiling method.

**Category:** A strongly effective gem water.

## Kunzite (Spodumene)

**Mineralogy:** Pink inosilicate of the pyroxene group (monocl., prim.)

**Indications:** Devotion, humility, promotes being true to oneself. Improves the memory and empathy; allows closeness with others. Encourages critical faculties, tolerance and the willingness to serve. Helps with neuralgia and ischial pain, toothache and impairment of the sensory organs; dissolves tensions in the area of the heart.

**Preparation:** All methods are suitable.

**Category:** A gently effective gem water.

## Labradorite (Feldspar)

**Mineralogy:** Feldspar with iridescent flashes (tectosilicate, tricl., prim.)

**Indications:** Imagination, creativity, depth of feeling, enthusiasm, wealth of ideas, reflection, truth. Revives forgotten memories and shows how things really are (dispels illusion). Reduces sensitivity to cold; helps with colds, rheumatism and gout. Has a calming and blood-pressure lowering effect.

**Preparation:** All methods are suitable.

**Category:** A strongly effective gem water.

## Labradorite, white (Feldspar, 'Rainbow Moonstone')

**Mineralogy:** Bluish-white Labradorite (triclinic, primary)

**Indications:** Sensitivity; the ability to feel and sense, good imagination, alertness, perceptiveness; seeing the world with amazement. Encourages intuition, mediumistic talent and artistic talent. Improves body image; regulates the female hormone cycle and helps with menstrual complaints.

**Preparation:** All methods are suitable.

**Category:** A strongly effective gem water.

## Lapis lazuli

**Mineralogy:** Lazurite rock (Lazurite: tectosilicate, cubic, tertiary)

**Indications:** Truth, honesty, dignity, friendship. Helps to offer criticism and receive it. Good for complaints of the throat, thyroid, larynx, vocal chords, nerves and the brain. Lapis lazuli without pyrite (golden inclusions) has the effect of lowering blood pressure; with pyrite it raises the blood pressure. Lengthens the menstrual cycle.

**Preparation:** All methods are suitable.

**Category:** An intensely effective gem water.

## Larimar (Blue Pectolite)

**Mineralogy:** Pectolite containing copper (inosilicate, tricl., prim.)

**Indications:** Openness, self-determination, responsibility. Widens scope spiritually; expands perception and helps work through impressions that have been absorbed. Encourages brain, nerve and sensory activity and helps with complaints affecting the head, throat and chest. Encourages growth in children.

**Preparation:** All methods are suitable.

**Category:** A strongly effective gem water.

## Lime Oolite (Roestone, Margarita stone)

**Mineralogy:** Crystal with chalk beads (trigonal/orthorhombic, sec.)

**Indications:** Purification, clarification, security, (gentle) strength. Liberates from spiritual ballast; protects against over-burdening; promotes sleep through the night. Encourages elimination, purifies, detoxifies; relieves headaches caused by metabolic problems. Strengthens the liver, stomach, intestines; lowers temperatures.

**Preparation:** All methods are suitable.

**Category:** A gently effective gem water.

## Magnesite

**Mineralogy:** Magnesium carbonate (trigonal, secondary)

**Indications:** Self-acceptance, relaxation, patience, compliance. Helps with stress, nervousness, anxiety, irritability. Detoxifies; lowers acidity, good for the stomach, intestine and gall bladder; helps with pain, tensions, colic, cramp, migraines, headaches, grinding of teeth, sore muscles, heartburn, nausea, pains in the limbs.

**Preparation:** All methods are suitable except the boiling method.

**Category:** A gently effective gem water.

## Magnetite

**Mineralogy:** Magnetic iron oxide (cubic, primary/tertiary)

**Indications:** Motivation, orientation, alignment of awareness. Increases the ability to react; stimulates one to measure usefulness and non-usefulness against higher ideals. Strengthens the liver and gall bladder; stimulates energy flow in the body; activates function of the glands (use regularly for a maximum of 1–2 weeks only).

**Preparation:** All methods are suitable except boiling and evaporation.

**Category:** An intensely effective gem water.

## Malachite

**Mineralogy:** Basic copper carbonate (monoclinic, secondary)
**Indications:** Intensity, curiosity, beauty, expression of feelings. Removes inhibitions; aids sexual difficulties. Stimulates the brain, nerves, liver, gall bladder; detoxifies; removes over-acidity; helps with cramp, nausea, vomiting, rheumatism, gout. Strengthens female reproductive organs; helps with menstrual problems; eases labour.
**Preparation:** Test tube method; conducting with crystals.
**Category:** An intensely effective gem water.

## Moldavite

**Mineralogy:** Glass formed by the impact of a meteorite (amorphous)
**Indications:** Freedom, detachment, no boundaries, space, spiritual generosity. Encourages remembering, dreaming and clairvoyance; draws one's attention from strong attachments and brings about the realization that one is a spiritual being. Helps with asthma, respiratory illnesses, influenza and anaemia; calms the nerves and senses.
**Preparation:** All methods are suitable.
**Category:** An intensely effective gem water.

## Mookaite

**Mineralogy:** Jasper Opal mixture (trigonal/amorphous, secondary)
**Indications:** Variety and fun, combines inner peace with spirit of adventure; helps process experiences. Strengthens the immune system and blood purification via the liver and spleen. Encourages wound healing; helps inflammations with pus. Strengthens the digestion; helps with stomach and intestinal complaints, nausea and constipation.
**Preparation:** All methods are suitable.
**Category:** A gently effective gem water.

## Moonstone (Feldspar)

**Mineralogy:** Feldspar with wavy glow (monoclinic, primary)
**Indications:** Intuition, depth of feeling, empathy, openness, perception. Encourages remembering dreams; helps with sleepwalking (take the gem water from the time of the New Moon); eases hormonal transitions (puberty, menstruation, pregnancy, after giving birth, menopause). Encourages fertility in women.
**Preparation:** All methods are suitable.
**Category:** Strongly effective; intensity greatest at the Full Moon!

## Moss Agate

**Mineralogy:** Chalcedony with green dendrites (trigonal, secondary)

**Indications:** Liberation, hope, inspiration. Dissolving of anxieties, pressure and burdens. Cleanses the connective tissues, mucous membranes and lymph glands. Helps with diabetes, influenza, colds, coughs, stubborn infections, pains in the limbs, fevers and over-sensitivity to changes in the weather.

**Preparation:** All methods are suitable.

**Category:** Strongly effective gem water; possible to take larger amounts.

## Moss Agate, pink

**Mineralogy:** Chalcedony with brown chlorite (trigonal, secondary)

**Indications:** Purity, openness, honesty, directness. Helps overcome blame, thoughts of revenge, argumentativeness, grudges, disgust, revulsion. Stimulates digestion and elimination; improves activity of the intestine and intestinal flora; alleviates inflammations of the stomach and intestine; helps with nausea, constipation, diarrhoea.

**Preparation:** All methods are suitable.

**Category:** A gently effective gem water.

## Nephrite

**Mineralogy:** Compacted Actinolite (inosilicate, monoclinic, tertiary)

**Indications:** Balance, harmony. Protects against external pressure and aggressiveness; bestows inner balance. Helps with complaints of the kidneys, urinary tract and bladder; regulates water balance; encourages the detoxification of bodily fluids and tissues. Good for ear complaints, such as tinnitus, and disturbances of the sense of balance.

**Preparation:** All methods are suitable.

**Category:** A gently effective gem water.

## Obsidian

**Mineralogy:** Volcanic glass (silicon oxide, amorphous, primary)

**Indications:** Self-discovery, awareness, integration of one's shadow side. Relieves shocks, blocks, anxiety, pain, tensions, constriction of blood vessels. Regulates body temperature, improves blood circulation, clotting and wound healing. One element of 'emergency' gem water.

**Preparation:** All methods are suitable; avoid the boiling method with gold-sheen, silver-sheen or rainbow obsidian.

**Category:** An intensely effective gem water.

## Ocean Jasper (Ocean Agate, Orbicular Jasper)

**Mineralogy:** Spherulitic Chalcedony (quartz, trigonal, primary)
**Indications:** Vitality, hope, renewal, regeneration, awareness of the breadth of possibilities and infinite possibilities, energy to act, creativity, improving one's life. Makes one positive, able to cope with burdens; composed; helps one solve conflicts; good for exhaustion; encourages good sleep. Strengthens the immune system; encourages detoxification and elimination; improves lymph flow, as well as supply to and elimination from all the body's cells, tissues and organs. Helps with migraines, diabetes, thyroid problems, allergies, neurodermatitis, influenza, colds, coughs, swollen lymph glands, oedemas, pains in the limbs, fevers, stubborn infections (bacterial, viral and fungal), inflammations, inflammatory conditions with the formation of pus, leg ulcers, cysts, fibroids and tumours and cancer. Good for the skin, mucous membranes, respiratory system, ears, eyes and hollow organs (stomach, intestines, bladder, prostate, uterus), kidneys, liver, gall bladder, prostate, testes and ovaries. Encourages fertility.
**Preparation:** All methods are suitable.
**Category:** A gently effective gem water.

## Onyx

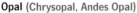

**Mineralogy:** Black Chalcedony (trigonal, primary/secondary)
**Indications:** Assertiveness, self-confidence, sense of responsibility. Promotes unemotional thinking, logic and control. Encourages the purification and elimination of waste products in the tissues; fortifies the immune system; helps with inner ear infections; sharpens the sense of hearing and improves the function of sensory and motor nerves.
**Preparation:** All methods are suitable.
**Category:** A gently effective gem water.

## Opal (Chrysopal, Andes Opal)

**Mineralogy:** Opal containing copper (silicon dioxide, amorphous, sec.)
**Indications:** Naturalness, openness, the ability to be enthusiastic. Frees feelings, lightens mood, helps one to see the world with amazement. Frees the heart and chest of feelings of oppression, detoxifies, stimulates the lymph system, lowers temperatures and relieves cramp; encourages the ability of the liver to regenerate.
**Preparation:** All methods are suitable except the boiling method.
**Category:** A strongly effective gem water.

## Opal (Pink Opal, Andes Opal)
**Mineralogy:** Opal containing manganese (silicon dioxide, am., sec.)
**Indications:** Warm-heartedness, uninhibited manner, carefreeness. Dissolves inhibitions, shame and shyness; encourages empathy and affection. Makes one friendly and open in one's thinking and actions; helps with heart problems, especially with worries about the heart (heart neuroses).
**Preparation:** All methods are suitable except the boiling method.
**Category:** A gently effective gem water.

## Opal, white (Milky Opal)
**Mineralogy:** White Opal (silicon dioxide, amorphous, prim./sec.)
**Indications:** Openness, flexibility, activity. Makes one open and accommodating; helps one to accept people and situations. Encourages communication, exchange and community. Stimulates cleansing of the skin, the respiratory organs and tissues; strengthens the kidneys, bladder, lymph flow and regulation of the body's water balance.
**Preparation:** All methods are suitable except the boiling method.
**Category:** A gently effective gem water.

## Opalite
**Mineralogy:** rock containing opal (Opal: amorphous, secondary)
**Indications:** Sociability; friendliness. Helps remove fear of physical contact; improves contact with one's environment and other people. Encourages detoxification and elimination; purifies the connective tissues, intestines and mucous membranes. Strengthens the lungs' capacity to absorb oxygen; helps with damage caused by smoking.
**Preparation:** All methods are suitable except the boiling method.
**Category:** A strongly effective gem water.

## Orthoclase (Feldspar, Gold Orthoclase)
**Mineralogy:** Potassium Feldspar (tectosilicate, monoclinic, primary)
**Indications:** Perception and good insightfulness. Makes one optimistic, exhilarated and full of joie de vivre; reduces worries, doubts and mistrust. Strengthens the sense of right action at the right time. Helps with nerve complaints, stomach complaints, heart problems, chest constriction, restlessness and sleeplessness.
**Preparation:** All methods are suitable.
**Category:** A gently effective gem water.

## Picture Jasper (Kalahari Picture Stone)

**Mineralogy:** Quartz sandstone (Jasper, trigonal, secondary)
**Indications:** Stamina, steadfastness, staying power, simplicity, humility. Good for the stomach, spleen, pancreas and intestine. Encourages digestion and elimination, boosts the immune system and cleansing of the connective tissues. Thus helpful with food intolerances, allergies and hay fever.
**Preparation:** All methods are suitable.
**Category:** A gently effective gem water.

## Peridot (Olivine)

**Mineralogy:** Magnesium iron nesosilicate (orthorhombic, primary)
**Indications:** Independence, purification. Dissolves anger and guilt; helps to detach from external influences, acknowledge mistakes and forgive. Stimulates detoxification and elimination (especially of fatty tissues); encourages liver, gall bladder, small intestine and metabolic function. Helps with skin problems, warts and fungal infections.
**Preparation:** All methods are suitable.
**Category:** An intensely effective gem water.

## Prase/Prase Quartz (Budstone)

**Mineralogy:** Quartz with green silicate inclusions (trigonal, primary)
**Indications:** Gentleness, serenity, self-control. Cools hot-headed people; eases the resolution of conflicts; lowers high temperatures; alleviates pain; effective for swellings, bruises and bladder problems. Helps with insect bites, sunburn, sunstroke, heatstroke and minor burns. In combination with Aventurine, good for psoriasis.
**Preparation:** All methods are suitable.
**Category:** A gently effective gem water.

## Precious Opal

**Mineralogy:** Opal with flashes of iridescence (amorphous, sec.)
**Indications:** Joie de vivre, imagination, sensuality, cheerfulness, wit, creativity. Helps with sorrow, homesickness; depression. Strengthens lymph flow and the immune system; eliminates waste; helps with respiratory illnesses. Keeps one young and healthy.
**Preparation:** Direct placing in water; test tube method (for Opals with the matrix still attached); conducting with crystals.
**Category:** A gently effective gem water.

## Prehnite
**Mineralogy:** Calcium aluminium phyllosilicate (orthorhombic, prim.)
**Indications:** Attention, respect, acceptance, acknowledgement. Helps with accepting oneself and others and accepting unpleasant truths. Dissolves mechanisms of suppression and avoidance. Encourages the dissolving of fat-soluble substances; stimulates the metabolism and renewal processes and helps with problems with overweight.
**Preparation:** All methods are suitable.
**Category:** A gently effective gem water.

## Rhodochrosite
**Mineralogy:** Pink to reddish manganese carbonate (trigonal, secondary)
**Indications:** Activity, liveliness, love, eroticism, sexuality, enthusiasm. Lightens mood; lends energy in cases of exhaustion. Stimulates the circulation, blood pressure, kidneys and sexual glands (testes and ovaries). Helps with migraines and abdominal problems. **Warning:** Only use for 1–2 weeks. Do not use if you have high blood pressure.
**Preparation:** All methods are suitable except the boiling method.
**Category:** An intensely effective gem water.

## Rhodonite
**Mineralogy:** Calcium manganese isosilicate (triclinic, tertiary)
**Indications:** Reconciliation, forgiveness, understanding, friendship. Makes it possible to let go of emotional burdens and emotional damage. Strengthens the heart, circulation, muscles, gums, stomach and blood vessels. Helps with haemorrhoids, injuries, contusions, pain, leg ulcers, autoimmune illnesses and multiple sclerosis.
**Preparation:** All methods (do not boil if black inclusions are present).
**Category:** A strongly effective gem water.

## Rose Quartz
**Mineralogy:** Rose-coloured quartz (silicon dioxide, trigonal, primary)
**Indications:** Warmth, love, empathy, directness, sensitivity, sensuality, romance. Makes one aware of one's own needs. Strengthens the heart, circulation, supply of blood to the tissues, reproductive organs; encourages fertility in women. Helps with sexual problems. Makes the skin soft and velvety.
**Preparation:** All methods are suitable.
**Category:** A gently effective gem water.

## Ruby

**Mineralogy:** Corundum containing chromium (trig., prim./usually tert.)
**Indications:** Passion, joie de vivre, bravery, virtue, courage. Bestows vibrancy, enthusiasm; encourages commitment and performance readiness. Warming and sexually stimulating. Strengthens the spleen, circulation, adrenal glands, reproductive organs; regulates blood pressure; improves blood circulation; brings out fevers if necessary.
**Preparation:** All methods are suitable.
**Category:** An intensely effective gem water.

## Rutilated Quartz

**Mineralogy:** Rutilated fibres in Quartz (tetragonal/trigonal, primary)
**Indications:** Independence, freedom, space, honesty, spiritual greatness. Mood-enhancing, antidepressant; liberates from feelings of oppression and anxiety. Loosens phlegm with coughs; helps with allergies, bronchitis, asthma, difficulties with breathing, the intestines and the heart. Good for growth, posture, the back and the spine.
**Preparation:** All methods are suitable.
**Category:** A gently effective gem water.

## Sapphire

**Mineralogy:** Corundum (trigonal, primary/usually tertiary)
**Indications:** Spiritual strength, sharp wit, love of truth, serenity. For unshakeable inner peace and all-encompassing love. Calms, brings clarity of thought and helps with depressions and delusions. Good for intestinal, brain and nerve illnesses; alleviates pain and lowers high temperatures and high blood pressure.
**Preparation:** All methods are suitable.
**Category:** An intensely effective gem water.

## Sard

**Mineralogy:** Brown Chalcedony (Quartz, trigonal, prim./secondary)
**Indications:** Emotional strength, steadfastness, helpfulness, goodness. Lends strength; helps to overcome burdening situations; helps overcome disappointments and to assist others with word and deed. Improves the circulation of the heart; very good for weak heart and heart rhythm disturbances. Helps with headaches and ear complaints.
**Preparation:** All methods are suitable.
**Category:** A gently effective gem water.

## Sardonyx

**Mineralogy:** Chalcedony/Sard/Onyx (trigonal, primary/secondary)

**Indications:** Virtue, friendliness, helpfulness. Intensifies perception; supports all the sensory organs; helps with tinnitus. Stimulates the lymph flow, blood circulation, the spleen and intestines. Strengthens the immune response; helps properly heal illnesses. Good for influenza, colds, sore throats, middle ear infections and pains in the limbs.

**Preparation:** All methods are suitable.

**Category:** A gently effective gem water.

## Serpentine

**Mineralogy:** Basal magnesium phyllosilicate (monoclinic, tertiary)

**Indications:** Peace, self-determination, protection. For nervousness, stress and sexual difficulties. Helps with sore muscles, injuries, sprains, pain, cramp, colic, menstrual disorders, migraine, heart rhythm disturbances, kidneys, stomach, gall bladder, intestinal complaints, excess acidity, diarrhoea and constipation.

**Preparation:** All methods (do not place 'silver-eye' in water).

**Category:** A gently effective gem water.

## Smoky Quartz

**Mineralogy:** Brown crystalline quartz (trigonal, primary)

**Indications:** Relaxation, stress reduction, ability to cope with burdens. Assists in tolerating anxiety, sorrow and exertion. Clarifies thinking; helps one be pragmatic. Helps with pain, tensions, intestinal problems and a weakened immune system caused by great strain. Strengthens the nerves; helps with working through the effects of radiation.

**Preparation:** All methods are suitable.

**Category:** A gently effective gem water.

## Sodalite

**Mineralogy:** Tectosilicate containing sodium (cubic, primary)

**Indications:** Awareness, striving for truth, idealism, being true to oneself. Good for the throat, larynx, vocal chords, kidneys and bladder. Has a cooling, fever-abating effect; regulates high blood pressure and water balance. In cases of dryness of eyes, skin and mucous membranes, it supports the absorption of fluids and the natural feeling of thirst.

**Preparation:** All methods are suitable.

**Category:** A gently effective gem water.

## Stromatolite

**Mineralogy:** Sediment formed by silicic algae (secondary)
**Indications:** Adaptability, ability to change, creative power. Encourages compliance, while retaining a firm point of view. Helps work through cumulated experiences and grow from them. Cleanses the connective tissues and the intestines; improves intestinal flora; encourages metabolism and elimination; dissolves abdominal tensions.
**Preparation:** All methods are suitable.
**Category:** A gently effective gem water.

## Sugilite

**Mineralogy:** Cyclosilicate containing minerals (hexagonal, primary)
**Indications:** Consistency, uncompromising attitude, resolution of conflicts. Lends the strength to remain true to oneself; to carry out intentions without faltering, and helps with anxieties and paranoia. Harmonizes nerves and brain; alleviates strong pain (even toothache) and helps with nervous complaints, dyslexia and motor disturbances.
**Preparation:** All methods are suitable.
**Category:** An intensely effective gem water.

## Sunstone (Aventurine **Feldspar**)

**Mineralogy:** Glittering brown Feldspar (tectosilicate, triclinic, primary)
**Indications:** Joie de vivre, positive attitude towards life, optimism, self-acceptance; lifting of mood, antidepressant; helps with anxieties and worries. Harmonizes the autonomic nervous system and the interaction of all the internal organs; strengthens metabolism and digestion; improves blood quality; stabilizes the circulation.
**Preparation:** All methods are suitable.
**Category:** An intensely effective gem water.

## Thulite (**Zoisite**)

**Mineralogy:** Zoisite containing manganese (sorosilicate, orthorhombic, tertiary)
**Indications:** Vitality, lust, sensuality. Bestows pleasure in sexuality. Encourages fertility and potency; helps with disorders of the reproductive organs. Aids regeneration in cases of exhaustion; blood formation and quality; blood cleansing in the liver and spleen.
**Preparation:** All methods are suitable.
**Category:** An intensely effective gem water.

## Tiger's Eye

**Mineralogy:** Yellowish-brown fibrous Quartz (trigonal, secondary)
**Indications:** Insight, detachment, sharpness of the senses. Helps with stress, burdens and with moods affected by external influences. Alleviates pain; regulates the adrenals and helps with acute asthma attacks (for this, transparent Tiger's Eye Quartz is best).

**Preparation:** Placing crystals directly in water; test tube method (with fibrous raw crystals); conducting with crystals.
**Category:** A gently effective gem water.

## Tiger Iron

**Mineralogy:** Hematite Jasper Tiger's Eye crystal (trigonal, tertiary)
**Indications:** Vitality, change, new beginnings. Helps to overcome difficulties and to find pragmatic solutions fast and decisively. Works quickly for exhaustion, circulatory problems and iron deficiency, encourages the formation of blood and a supply of oxygen to all cells and organs.

**Preparation:** Test tube method; conducting with crystals.
**Category:** A strongly effective gem water.

## Topaz, blue

**Mineralogy:** Light blue aluminium nesosilicate (orthorhombic, prim.)
**Indications:** Self-realization, self-trust, inner riches, wisdom through life's experience. Strengthens the nerves, digestion and metabolism and raises the energy flow in the meridians. Helps with poor sight, stomachache, stomach and intestinal complaints, loss of weight and eating disorders (also sometimes with anorexia).

**Preparation:** All methods are suitable.
**Category:** Strongly effective; possible to take larger amounts.

## Topaz, imperial (Golden Topaz)

**Mineralogy:** Nesosilicate containing phosphorus (orthorhombic, prim.)
**Indications:** Self-realization, self-confidence, self-worth. Generosity, charisma, a positive attitude; relieves depression; for confidence, courage and success. Strengthens the nerves, stomach, pancreas, small intestine; stimulates appetite; helps with disturbances in growth, digestion and eating (anorexia). Encourages fertility in women.

**Preparation:** All methods are suitable.
**Category:** An intensely effective gem water.

**Tourmaline, black (Schorl)**
**Mineralogy:** Black iron aluminium Tourmaline (trigonal, primary)
**Indications:** Composure, neutrality, protection. Helps to ward off negative influences. Improves sleep; alleviates effects of radiation, stress, pain, tensions, joint problems and sensations of numbness. Encourages reduction of scarring and energy flow in the meridians. Helps with intestinal complaints, flatulence and constipation.
**Preparation:** All methods are suitable except the boiling method.
**Category:** Strongly effective; possible to take larger amounts.

**Tourmaline, blue (Indigolite)**
**Mineralogy:** Blue Tourmaline (boron cyclosilicate, trigonal, pimary)
**Indications:** Loyalty, ethics, responsibility, tolerance, striving for spiritual freedom. Releases tears and held-in feelings. Helps with hyperactivity and disturbances in growth and development. Strengthens the nerves, eyes, kidneys, bladder and water balance. Helps with burns (with Chrysocolla); joint problems; sensations of numbness.
**Preparation:** All methods are suitable except the boiling method.
**Category:** Strongly effective; possible to take large amounts.

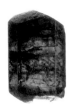

**Tourmaline, brown (Dravite)**
**Mineralogy:** Magnesium aluminium Tourmaline (trigonal, primary)
**Indications:** Sense of community, helpfulness, social commitment. Helps give up compulsive behaviour and damaging habits. Strengthens the stomach; alleviates over-acidity; stimulates the regeneration of the skin, cells and tissues; helps with cellulite and growth disturbances and promotes the healing of scars.
**Preparation:** All methods are suitable except the boiling method.
**Category:** Strongly effective; possible to take larger amounts.

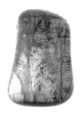

**Tourmaline, green (Verdelite)**
**Mineralogy:** Green Tourmaline (boron cyclosilicate, trigonal, primary)
**Indications:** Interest, gratitude, openness, patience. Helps with hyperactivity, nervous complaints (in this case, use Watermelon Tourmaline with a pink centre enfolded in green), rheumatism, degenerative processes and tumours. Strengthens the eyes, heart, intestine, elimination and joints; detoxifies and helps to reduce scarring.
**Preparation:** All methods are suitable except the boiling method.
**Category:** Strongly effective; possible to take larger amounts.

## Tourmaline, red (Rubellite)

**Mineralogy:** Red Tourmaline (boron cyclosilicate, trigonal, primary)
**Indications:** Liveliness, joy, compassion, thirst for adventure, sociability, charm. Brings spiritual warmth; encourages sexuality. Strengthens the nerves, blood, spleen, liver, heart, reproductive organs. Helps with weakness of the optic nerve, and with joint problems resulting in lack of energy and sensations of numbness in the limbs.
**Preparation:** All methods are suitable except the boiling method.
**Category:** Strongly effective; possible to take larger amounts.

## Tourmaline Quartz

**Mineralogy:** Tourmaline needles (Schorl) in Quartz (trigonal, primary)
**Indications:** Balance, harmony, connecting polarities. Helps release inner struggles and conflicts, as well harmonizing opposites. Balances excess energy and lack of energy; strengthens the nerves; eases tensions, cramp, hardening of muscles; keeps one lively and mobile; encourages cleansing and elimination.
**Preparation:** All methods are suitable.
**Category:** A gently effective gem water.

## Turquoise

**Mineralogy:** Basal copper aluminium phosphate (triclinic, secondary)
**Indications:** Self-determination, responsibility, protection. Balances mood swings. Good for asthma, ear infections (also tinnitus), over-acidity, heartburn, nausea, menstrual problems, rheumatism, gout. Has a pain-alleviating effect; eases cramp; calms inflammations; fortifies the brain, liver and stomach.
**Preparation:** Test tube method; conducting with crystals.
**Category:** A strongly effective gem water.

## Zoisite

**Mineralogy:** Calcium aluminium sorosilicate (orthorhombic, tertiary)
**Indications:** Building up, regeneration, creativity, spiritual fulfilment. Aids recovery after illnesses or severe stress. Alleviates inflammations; detoxifies; balances over-acidity; strengthens the immune system, liver and kidneys. Promotes fertility; helps with diseases of the prostate, testes and ovaries. Zoisite with ruby increases potency.
**Preparation:** All methods are suitable
**Category:** A gently effective gem water.

## The authors

### Michael Gienger

Michael Gienger thinks of himself as a naturalist. For him Nature is just one great book, in which the many mysteries of life can be recognized and understood through observation and awareness. He is self-taught and has earned international acclaim with his contributions to crystal healing. His research activity does, however, cover the entire vast field of nature study and natural healing. The subject of water especially has fascinated him since his youth. In the introduction to his first book, 'Crystal Power, Crystal Heal-

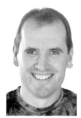

ing', which was first published in German in 1995, he wrote, 'Among my earliest memories are those of stones, inseparably linked in my mind with running water, and mountain streams in particular. I loved to divert the flow of the water with the aid of dams built with large and small pebbles.' Both crystal healing and knowledge about water have become firm elements of his research and activities over the last 20 years. This new book at last brings together both of his 'great' research areas, in order to provide a firm basis for a new branch of crystal healing.

You will find more about Michael Gienger and his projects on the internet under www.steinheilkunde.de, www.michael-gienger.de, wwww.fairtrademinerals.de, and wwww.cairn-elen.de among others.

### Joachim Goebel

Joachim Goebel, too, was a 'water child'; even in early childhood, he was always irresistibly drawn to the water element. Playful activities with water deepened into natural curiosity in his youth, and he became increasingly interested in the study of this natural phenomenon. His interest in healing grew steadily at the same time. Joachim Goebel studied medicine and then dedicated himself, in parallel, to Ayurvedic studies and various different natural healing processes. In this connection he recognized water as the

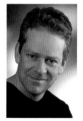

elixir of life in this, our mortal state, and he devoted himself with even greater commitment to the holistic research of water. In 1997, he was introduced to the subject of crystal healing. Further inspired by the teachings of the medieval naturalist Hildegard von Bingen, Joachim Goebel began his 'water and gem' research in 1998. At the time, gem water was largely unheard of, so he began with initial examinations and trials. They were so successful that the subject of gem water became the focus of his daily professional activities. As a lecturer in crystal healing he gives talks, seminars and training on the subject of gem water and also offers personal consultations.

More on Joachim Goebel and his projects can be found on the internet under www.edelstein-wasser.de. The authors also publish supplements to this book and more recent results on their websites.

## Picture credits

Ines Blersch: all photographs, except following ones:
  Dragon Design: p. 38 bottom; Ruth Kübler: p. 28; Vita-Juwel: p. 42 top, 44, 45 top; Josef Zerluth: p. 7

## Bibliography

Michael Gienger, *The Healing Crystal First Aid Manual, A practical A to Z of common ailments and illnesses and how they can be best treated with crystal therapy*, published by Earthdancer, a Findhorn Press Imprint, in 2006

Michael Gienger, *Crystal Power Crystal Healing*, published by Cassell Illustrated in 1998

Michael Gienger, *Healing Crystals, The A-Z Guide to 430 Gemstones*, published by Earthdancer, a Findhorn Press Imprint, in 2005

## Continuing research on Gem Water

Research into the manufacture, compatibility and application of gem water is still in its infancy. If you have any questions, or you wish for more information or to read more reports on experiences with gem water, please refer to the following sources:

### Crystall-Quelle
Joachim Goebel
Nägeleseestr. 25
D-79102 Freiburg
Tel (0)761 707 69 40
info@ edelsteinwasser.de
www.edelsteinwasser.de

## Gem Authenticity Checks

Specialist laboratory for examining and checking authenticity of gems and minerals:

### Institut für Edelstein-prüfung (EPI)
(Gem Authenticity Research Institute)
Riesenwaldstr. 6
D-77797 Ohlsbach
Tel (0) 7803 600 808
lab@epigem.de
www.epigem.de

## Crystal Healing

### Research; public relations; consumer protection

Steinheilkunde e.V.,
Registered seat:
Stuttgart
Forschungsprojekt
Steinheilkunde
(Crystal Healing
Research Project)
Hildener Str. 40
D-42329 Wuppertal
Tel (0) 202 317 67 512
info@steinheilkunde-
  ev.de
www.steinheilkunde-
  ev.de

## Seminars and training

### Cairn Elen Lebens-schule Tübingen
Annette Jakobi
Mozartstrasse 9
D-72127 Kusterdingen
Tel (0)7071 538 266
annette@edelsteinmas
  sagen.de
www.edelstein-massag
  en.de/tuebingen

### Cairn Elen Lebens-schule Schwä. Alb
Dagmar Fleck
Rossgumpenstrasse 10
D-72336 Balingen
Tel (0)7435 919 932
info@cairn-elen.de
www.cairn-elen.de

### Cairn Elen Lebens-schule Nürnberg
Petra Endres
Kleiststrasse 4
D-90491 Nürnberg
Tel (0) 911 598 87 29
info@petra-endres.de
www.petra-endres.de

### Freiburger Stein-heilkunde-Schule Crystal-Balance
Joachim Goebel
Nägeleseestr. 25
D-79102 Freiburg
Tel (0)761 707 69 40
info@crystall-quelle.de
www.crystall-balance.de

### Akademie Lapis Vitalis
Im Osterholz 1
D-71636 Ludwigsburg
Tel (0) 7141 4412 88
info@lapisvitalis.de
www.lapisvitalis.de

This is an easy-to-use A-Z guide for treating many common ailments and illnesses with the help of crystal therapy. It includes a comprehensive colour appendix with photographs and short descriptions of each gemstone recommended.

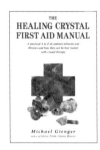

Michael Gienger

**The Healing Crystal First Aid Manual**

A Practical A to Z of Common Ailments and Illnesses and How They Can Be Best Treated with Crystal Therapy

*288 pages, with 16 colour plates*

ISBN 978-1-84409-084-6

This book introduces a spectrum of massage possibilities using healing crystals. The techniques have been developed and refined by experts, and this wisdom is conveyed in simple and direct language, enhanced by photos. Any interested amateur will be amazed at the wealth of new therapeutic possibilities that open up when employing the healing power of crystals.

Michael Gienger

**Crystal Massage for Health and Healing**

*112 pages, full colour throughout*

ISBN 978-1-84409-077-8

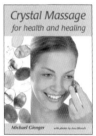

For further information and book catalogue contact:
Findhorn Press, 117-121 High Street, Forres, IV36 1AB, Scotland.
Earthdancer Books is an imprint of Findhorn Press.
tel +44 (0)1309-690582  fax +44 (0)1309-690036
info@findhornpress.com  www.earthdancer.co.uk  www.findhornpress.com

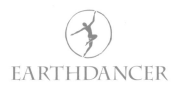

EARTHDANCER

A FINDHORN PRESS IMPRINT